To. Mum
with lots of love
from
( )

HIGH-FIBRE
COOKERY

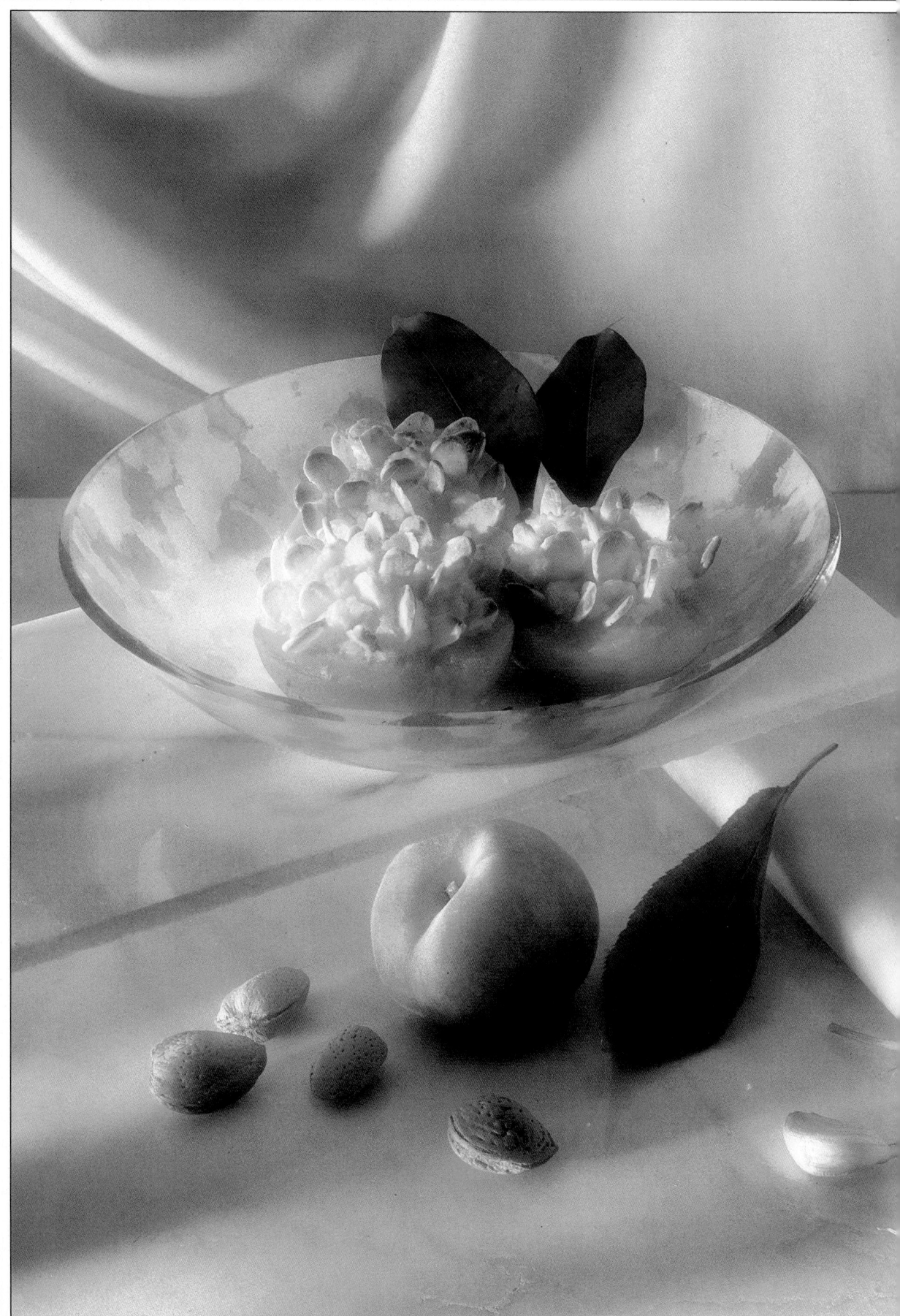

RECIPES FOR GOOD HEALTH

HIGH-FIBRE
COOKERY

Written and compiled by
Alison Leach and Jane Lewis, SRD

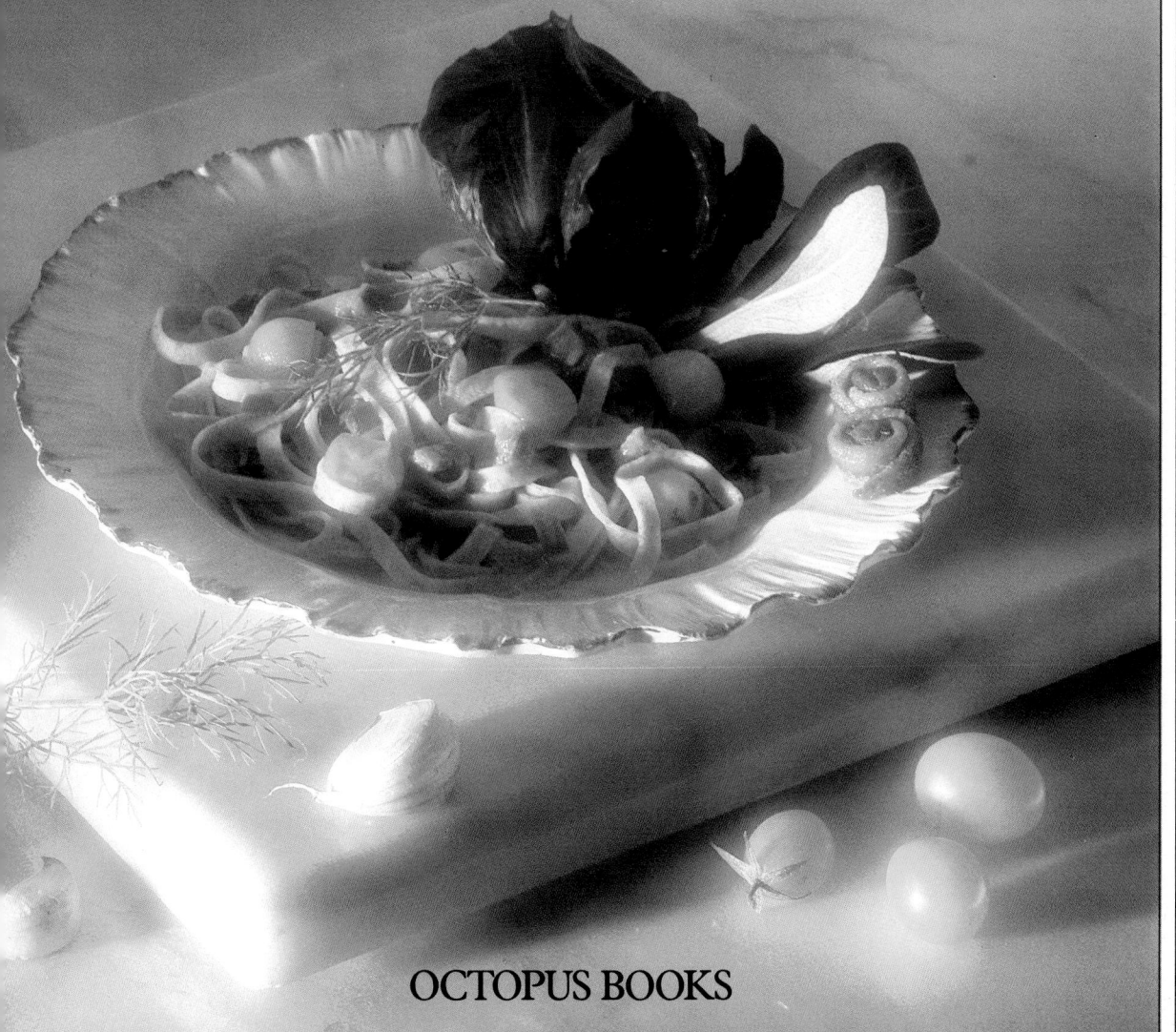

OCTOPUS BOOKS

ACKNOWLEDGMENTS

The publisher acknowledges the following photographers: Bryce Attwell page 71; Robert Golden pages 43, 46–7, 49, 57; Melvin Grey pages 11, 15, 34, 83; Gina Harris pages 64, 66–7; Roger Phillips pages 104, 108–9, 112, 116; Grant Symon cover, pages 2–3, 21, 24–5, 52–3, 78–9, 94–5, 100–1; Paul Williams pages 17, 35, 38–9, 42, 60–1. Brittany Prince Artichokes provided the photograph on page 75, the Kellogg Company of Great Britain the photograph on page 91, the Mushroom Growers' Association the photograph on page 86 and the White Fish Kitchen the photograph on page 29. Cookware, dishes and cutlery used in Grant Symon's photography were supplied by: Elizabeth David, 46 Bourne Street, London SW1; Graham and Green, 4 & 7 Elgin Crescent, London W11; Smash and Grab, 662 Fulham Road, London SW6; and Joanna Wood, 48A Pimlico Road, London SW1.

Line drawings by Alun Jones.

Cover illustration: Autumn slaw (page 62), Devilled turkey kebabs with apricot pilaff (page 72), Orange sorbet with raspberries (page 114). Title spread illustration: Spiced stuffed peaches (page 107), Noodles with anchovy sauce (page 88).

Much of the information in the section Fibre content of foods, pages 124–5, is derived from *The Composition of Foods* by R.A. McCance and E.M. Widdowson, 4th edition, 1978, published by the British Medical Research Council and H.M.S.O.

COOKING NOTE

The measurements in the recipes are given in both metric and imperial units. Use whichever system you are familiar with, but do not mix the two as the equivalents are not exact.

When spoonfuls are mentioned use level spoons:
1 teaspoon = 5 ml,
1 tablespoon = 15 ml.

Australian readers who use a 20 ml tablespoon should use 3 × 5 ml teaspoons to get the correct measure for the recipes in this book.

A Ridgmount book

This edition first published 1986 by
Octopus Books Ltd
59 Grosvenor Street, London W1

ISBN 0 7064 2622 3

Printed in Hong Kong

CONTENTS

WHY HIGH FIBRE?

A diet rich in fibre is now considered by doctors and nutritionists throughout the world to be one of the best means of maintaining good health and of lessening the possibility of developing many of the disorders and illnesses prevalent in the Western world today.

This book shows how easily an enjoyable and attractive high-fibre diet can be created and offers a wide selection of over 200 tempting nutritious dishes to choose from.

FIBRE AND YOUR HEALTH

The fibrous substance forming the rigid structure of plant cell walls provides our source of dietary fibre. Because this fibre remains undigested as it passes through the intestine it was thought for many years to be unnecessary in our diet, and removing it was considered to improve the quality of food – hence the production of white bread with the fibre-rich husk of the wheat grains discarded.

Now it is realized that fibre exerts its beneficial effect in part by reducing the time taken for waste to pass through the digestive system. In addition, researchers have discovered that undigested fibre produces beneficial biochemical effects in the large bowel, as well as other positive metabolic changes. This type of fibre is known as insoluble fibre.

Recent research has shown that a second kind of fibre, soluble fibre, can help to reduce high blood sugar and cholesterol levels, the latter being a major factor in the development of coronary heart disease. The main sources of this fibre are oats and pulses, such as beans, peas and lentils.

Statistics show that intake of both types of fibre in many Third World countries is much higher than in Britain, the United States, Australia and other Western nations. The fact that many diseases prevalent in Western society are least common in Third World countries adds considerable weight to the widely accepted medical opinion that the high incidence of these Western disorders is directly related to low fibre and high fat intake. These ailments include: constipation, diverticular disease, appendicitis, piles (haemorrhoids), cancer of the large bowel, coronary heart disease, venous thrombosis, gallstones, diabetes and obesity.

GUIDELINES FOR A HEALTHY DIET

The need for Western societies to move towards a Third-World-type pattern of eating was highlighted in 1983 by the report published in Britain by the National Advisory Committee on Nutrition Education (NACNE). This report stressed the importance to good health of altering the contents of the average diet by increasing daily intake of fibre and lowering consumption of fat and sugar. It also recommended that the use of salt should be reduced substantially.

FIBRE You should aim to increase your fibre intake to an average of at least 30 g per day. The fibre content of all the book's recipes, which incorporate a large variety of high-fibre ingredients, is displayed in grams per portion. Using these figures and the information in the fibre content table at the end of the book, it is possible to plan and check your day's fibre intake.

FAT The energy content of foods is measured in kilocalories (kcal) – also popularly called calories – or kilojoules (kJ). Gram for gram, fat contains almost twice the calories of the other main constituents of food – protein and carbohydrate. The proportion of fat in the diet should be reduced from the present Western average of 40 per cent of total calories per day to 30 per cent. To help you achieve this we have included the fat value of each recipe in grams per portion. Remember that 1 g fat is the equivalent of 9 kcal/38 kJ. Recommended maximum fat intakes for the various daily calorie levels are as follows:

DAILY ENERGY INTAKE	MAXIMUM FAT
1500 kcal/6300 kJ	50 g
2000 kcal/8400 kJ	67 g
2500 kcal/10500 kJ	83 g
3000 kcal/12600 kJ	100 g

There are two types of fat: saturated and unsaturated. Almost all foods contain some fat but it is the saturated fats, found mainly in foods of animal origin, such as meat, milk, lard, butter and cheese which you should limit in particular.

The fat content of all this book's recipes has been kept to a minimum, with the high-fat foods such as cream, whole milk and full-fat cheese being replaced by lower-fat alternatives such as low-fat yogurt, skimmed milk and the lower-fat cheeses.

An overall reduction of fat in the diet and the replacement of saturated fats with un-saturated alternatives, such as vegetable oils and margarines high in polyunsat-urates, are considered to be important steps to help prevent heart disease. But bear in mind that saturated and unsaturated fats are equally high in calories.

If you choose one of the recipes with a comparatively high fat content, try to compensate by eating food with less fat at other meals to achieve a sensible overall balance for the day.

LOSING WEIGHT ON A HIGH-FIBRE DIET

Being overweight is known to be a risk factor to health, as it may lead to the development of one or more major ail-ments, including high blood pressure, coronary heart disease and diabetes.

You will put on weight if your calorie intake exceeds you calorie, or energy, requirements. Your lifestyle, age and sex determine your own particular energy re-quirements. A sportsman, for example, will need more energy than an office worker sitting at his desk all day.

Often the main culprits are calorie-rich foods high in sugar and fat but low in fibre, which do not leave you feeling satisfied. Fibre-rich foods tend to be lower in cal-ories and yet make you feel fuller and less hungry. So increasing your fibre intake really is useful if you are trying to lose weight. A combination of regular, well-balanced meals, low in sugar and fat but high in fibre, provides a sensible, healthy way of losing those excess pounds, and is far more likely to succeed in the long term than crash dieting.

Each recipe in this book has its energy content displayed in kcal/kJ per portion. If you are controlling your calorie intake, this will enable you to select recipes which suit your particular needs.

In addition, some of the calorie-counted meal plans at the end of the book have been specially created to help those trying to lose weight.

SOURCES OF FIBRE

Fibre is found only in foods of plant origin. This large family of foods can be divided into three groups: cereals, pulses, and fruit and vegetables.

CEREALS Whole grain cereals in which the fibre-rich husk remains intact are good sources of fibre. They should be used instead of processed cereals from which the fibre has been extracted during milling. Wherever possible 100 per cent stone-ground wholemeal flour should be used for making bread, pastry, cakes and biscuits.

Brown rice should be used instead of white; it takes slightly longer to cook and does not become soft, having a crunchier texture.

Wholemeal pasta is now available in a variety of shapes and sizes from many large supermarkets and health food shops. It takes a little longer to cook than pasta made with white flour but the result is well worth the few extra minutes' cooking time.

PULSES These include beans, peas and lentils. As well as being a good source of fibre, they are rich in protein and are used as protein foods in many vegetarian recipes.

A wide variety of pulses is now available, sold in either dried or canned form. Beans include the colourful kidney, aduki, mung and black-eye varieties. There are split orange lentils as well as whole green or brown ones. Dried peas range from the traditional dried whole green kind to the split golden yellow ones.

FRUIT AND VEGETABLES A superb variety of more exotic fruit and vegetables is now sold in our shops, providing a wide range of textures, flavours and colours.

As much of the fibre is contained in their skins, these should be left on wherever possible. It is therefore essential that fruit and vegetables should always be washed thoroughly before use.

Potatoes can be baked in their jackets or boiled or steamed in their skins. No fibre is lost and they are much better nutritionally than when cooked in fat.

Fruit and vegetable purées should be prepared in a blender so that the skins and pips can be included.

EATING THE HIGH-FIBRE WAY

If high-fibre cooking is new to you and those you cook for, it may be most successful if you introduce high-fibre foods into your diet slowly, gradually increasing the number of high-fibre dishes you serve rather than suddenly adopting a completely new eating pattern.

The sample meal plans on pages 122–3 show how different recipes can be combined in a well-balanced way. These suggestions show how much variety a high-fibre diet can offer and how broad the scope is for the health-conscious cook.

HIGH-FIBRE COOKING

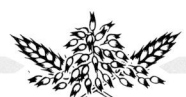

Eating should always be a source of enjoyment. This is the prime factor in making your family respond enthusiastically to a healthier high-fibre eating pattern. To help them make the change, you might like to try some of the family favourites in this book which have been given a high-fibre content, before introducing the more unusual recipes.

Other dishes are also very suitable to serve when entertaining friends who may not be familiar with high-fibre cooking.

Always serve crusty wholemeal rolls with main meals if the fat content is a little high. Do not put any butter or other type of fat on the table. Equally, try to dissuade your family from automatically adding salt to their food. Salt has not been included in the recipes in this book, but you may wish to add a little to them at first, gradually cutting out the salt as your family becomes used to the slightly different taste.

Develop their resistance to sugary desserts by substituting the natural sweetness of ripe fruit. Some of the recipies in the chapter on Desserts contain no added sugar.

Bread for sandwiches does not have to be spread with butter or margarine; try instead our recipes for Date spread or Crunchy peanut butter. Alternatively, choose fillings with a creamy texture, not ones that are too moist as they would make the bread soggy.

HEALTHY COOKING HINTS

- Use fresh wholemeal breadcrumbs instead of grated cheese for toppings.
- Thicken the liquid in a casserole with rolled oats instead of *beurre manié* (butter and flour) or a thickening agent.
- Make vegetable purées instead of rich sauces to serve with fish and poultry.
- Blend unsweetened fruit purées with plain unsweetened yogurt instead of buying flavoured varieties.
- Stabilize plain unsweetened yogurt to use in cooking instead of cream. To do this, mix 1 tablespoon cornflour with a little skimmed milk to form a paste. Stir it into 1 litre/1¾ pints yogurt, taking care to stir in one direction only. Bring the mixture to the boil slowly, and simmer, uncovered, for about 8 minutes or until it thickens. There will then be no risk of the yogurt curdling.
- Wipe the surplus oil or brine from canned tuna and other fatty fish with paper towels.
- Drain surplus fat from grilled bacon on absorbent kitchen paper.
- Allow stock to become cold so that the fat solidifies and can easily be removed from the surface.
- Remove as much fat as possible from meat before cooking.
- Use absorbent kitchen paper to absorb surplus oil when pre-cooking onions or other vegetables in a frying pan.
- Grill, bake or steam food rather than fry it.
- Most pulses should be soaked in cold water overnight. It is essential that red kidney beans and soya beans in particular are boiled rapidly for 10 minutes before simmering or adding to other ingredients in a casserole. The harmful enzymes in the beans are thus eliminated and the beans will then be perfectly safe to eat.
- The fibre content of foods is not affected by any cooking process, so there is considerabe scope for changing the texture to add variety. But it is best to avoid using a sieve as some of the fibre could be left behind and wasted.
- An extra-heavy frying pan with a non-stick coating is necessary to minimize the amount of fat used when pre-cooking vegetables or making griddlecakes.
- A range of non-stick cake tins and baking sheets is useful. Other tins should be lined with non-stick silicone paper. If it is impractical to line a tin, rub a little vegetable oil sparingly over the surface.
- Cut down on your fat intake by changing to skimmed or semi-skimmed milk and low-fat soft and reduced-fat hard cheeses.
- It is best to choose unshelled nuts as these will not have been salted or roasted in saturated fats.

Soups

ROOT VEGETABLE SOUP WITH LOVAGE

2 tablespoons olive oil
1 medium onion, thinly sliced
175 g/6 oz carrots, thinly sliced
175 g/6 oz parsnips, thinly sliced
175 g/6 oz turnips, thinly sliced
1 litre/1¾ pints chicken stock
freshly ground black pepper
4 tablespoons plain unsweetened yogurt
3 tablespoons chopped lovage

SERVES 4
Per serving: **Energy** 120 kcal/510 kJ
              Fat   8 g
              Fibre   5 g

Heat the oil and fry the onion gently, adding the other vegetables after 4 minutes. Cook gently for a further 8 minutes, then add the heated stock. Season to taste with pepper and simmer, covered, for 30 minutes, or until the vegetables are soft.

Purée briefly in a blender, or push through a medium food mill, and return to the pan. Reheat, adjust the seasoning and stir in the yogurt. Stir in the chopped lovage and stand the soup for a few moments before serving.

BLACK BEAN SOUP

125 g/5 oz black beans, soaked overnight in
   cold water
1.2 litres/2 pints cold water
1 celery stick, diced
1 medium onion, chopped
1 tablespoon dry sherry
freshly ground black pepper

TO GARNISH
1 hard-boiled egg, thinly sliced
1 lemon, thinly sliced

SERVES 4
Per serving: **Energy** 135 kcal/565 kJ
              Fat   2 g
              Fibre   5 g

Drain the beans and put in a saucepan with the cold water. Bring to the boil and cook rapidly for 10 minutes. Reduce the heat and add the celery and onion. Cover and simmer for about 1¼ hours until tender. The time will depend on how long the beans have been soaked. If necessary, add more water. Purée in a blender until smooth. Return the soup to the saucepan, add the sherry and season with pepper. Bring to the boil. Garnish each portion with slices of egg and lemon.

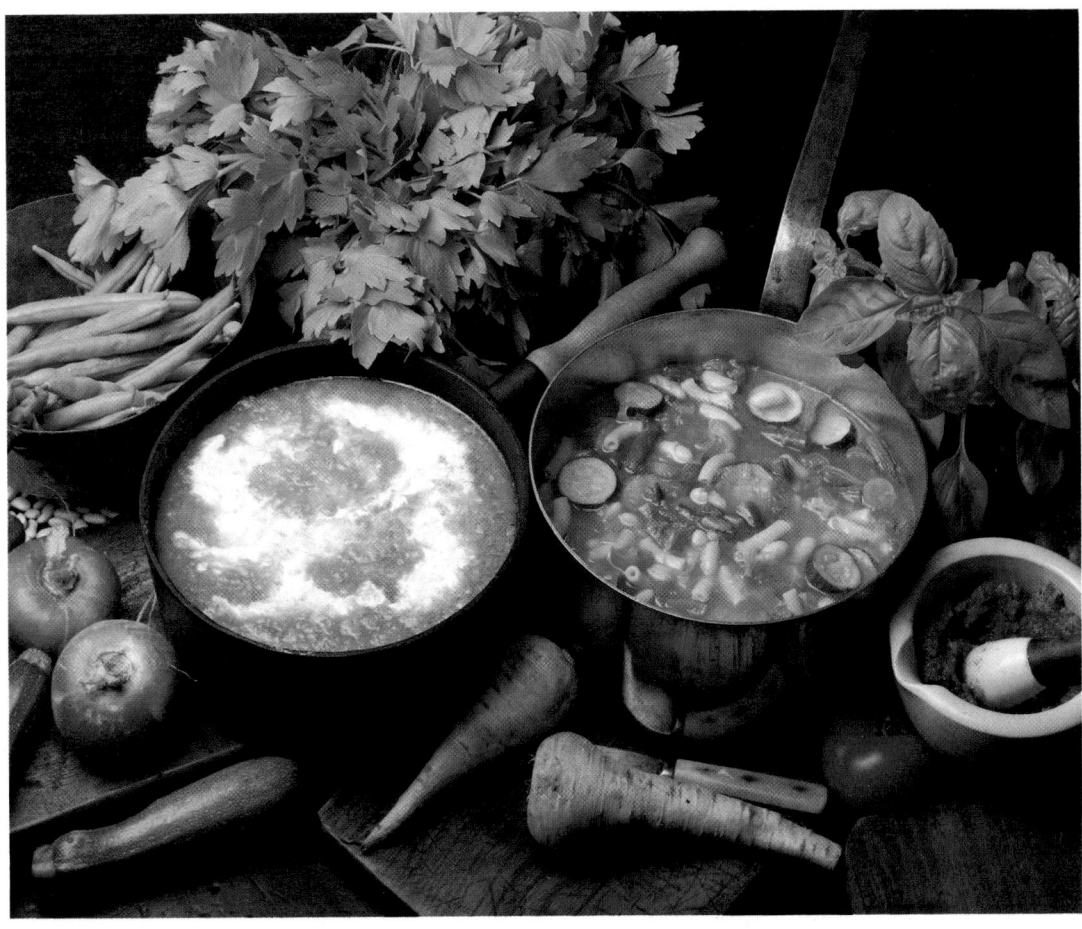

LEFT: ROOT VEGETABLE SOUP WITH LOVAGE;
RIGHT: MEDITERRANEAN VEGETABLE SOUP WITH PISTOU (P.41)

SPINACH SOUP

1 tablespoon olive oil
1 medium onion, chopped
2 × 225 g (8 oz) packets frozen chopped
   spinach
225 g/8 oz potatoes, peeled and diced
900 ml/1½ pints chicken stock
freshly ground black pepper
pinch of grated nutmeg
1 teaspoon lemon juice

300 ml/½ pint plain unsweetened yogurt,
   stabilized (page 9)
TO GARNISH
wholemeal croûtons

SERVES 4
Per serving: **Energy** 155 kcal/650 kJ
          Fat   6 g
          Fibre 6 g

Heat the oil in a saucepan and add the onion. Cook gently until soft. Add the spinach and heat through gently until thawed. Stir in the potatoes, stock, pepper to taste, nutmeg and lemon juice. Bring to the boil, cover and simmer gently for about 20 minutes or until the potato is breaking up. If a smooth soup is preferred, liquidize the mixture. Return to the pan, taste and adjust the seasoning and stir in the yogurt. Reheat gently. Serve with oven-baked croûtons.

WATERCRESS SOUP

300 g/11 oz cooked potatoes, chopped
750 ml/1¼ pints chicken stock
120 g/4½ oz watercress
freshly ground black pepper
TO GARNISH
sprigs watercress

SERVES 4
Per serving: **Energy** 70 kcal/295 kJ
             Fat negligible
             Fibre 3 g

Purée the potatoes, stock and watercress in a blender until smooth. Season with pepper. Put into a saucepan and bring to the boil, stirring frequently.

Serve the soup garnished with fresh watercress sprigs.

TOMATO SOUP

1 tablespoon olive oil
1 medium onion, finely chopped
100 g/4 oz peeled potatoes, thinly sliced
750 g/1½ lb ripe tomatoes, quartered
300 ml/½ pint water
1 small bay leaf
2 teaspoons tomato purée
150 ml/¼ pint skimmed milk

freshly ground black pepper
TO GARNISH
chopped fresh thyme

SERVES 4
Per serving: **Energy** 100 kcal/420 kJ
             Fat 4 g
             Fibre 4 g

Heat the oil in a saucepan and cook the onion over a low heat until soft. Add the potatoes, tomatoes, water, bay leaf and tomato purée. Simmer for about 20 minutes until the potatoes are cooked. Discard the bay leaf. Purée the mixture in a blender until smooth, then return to the saucepan. Add the milk and season with pepper. Bring to the boil, stirring frequently. Serve garnished with chopped thyme.

OATY VEGETABLE SOUP

1 tablespoon olive oil
1 medium onion, finely chopped
1 medium carrot, scrubbed and chopped
1 small turnip, peeled and chopped
1 leek, white and pale green part, washed and
    chopped
25 g/1 oz medium oatmeal
600 ml/1 pint stock

freshly ground black pepper
1 teaspoon chopped parsley
450 ml/¾ pint skimmed milk

SERVES 4
Per serving: **Energy** 125 kcal/520 kJ
             Fat 5 g
             Fibre 3 g

Heat the oil in a saucepan. Add the prepared vegetables and stir over gentle heat until all the oil is absorbed. Cover the pan and 'sweat' the vegetables for 2–3 minutes. Add the oatmeal and stir over moderate heat for a further 3–4 minutes. Pour on the stock, stir well and bring to the boil. Reduce the heat and simmer, covered, for 45 minutes. Season to taste and add the parsley.

Heat the milk in another saucepan until almost boiling. Stir into the soup and adjust the seasoning if necessary. Serve piping hot.

PUMPKIN SOUP WITH BASIL

450 g / 1 lb pumpkin, peeled and cut into 2 cm /
    1 inch cubes
225 g / 8 oz carrots, scrubbed and thinly sliced
900 ml / 1½ pints chicken stock
1 tablespoon olive oil
1 medium onion, chopped
225 g / 8 oz tomatoes, coarsely chopped
freshly ground black pepper

pinch of caster sugar
2 tablespoons chopped fresh basil

SERVES 4
Per serving: **Energy** 75 kcal / 305 kJ
               Fat 4 g
               Fibre 3 g

Put the pumpkin and the carrots in a pan with the stock and bring to the boil. Simmer, covered, for 20 minutes, or until soft.

Heat the oil in a saucepan and cook the onion gently for 4–5 minutes. Add the tomatoes and cook gently for 6 minutes, until slightly mushy.

Purée the pumpkin and carrots briefly in a blender, reserving about 300 ml / ½ pint of the liquid. Add as much of the reserved liquid as is needed to give a consistency of single cream. Stir in the onion and tomato mixture with its juice. Add pepper, a pinch of sugar and the basil. Stand, covered, for 5 minutes.

CARROT AND BANANA SOUP

225 g / 8 oz carrots, scrubbed and finely chopped
600 ml / 1 pint cold water
450 ml / ¾ pint chicken stock
3 medium bananas, peeled
freshly ground black pepper

SERVES 4
Per serving: **Energy** 60 kcal / 220 kJ
               Fat negligible
               Fibre 4 g

Put the carrots and water in a saucepan, bring to the boil and simmer until tender. Add the stock and bananas and bring back to the boil. Purée in a blender until smooth. Season with pepper. This soup may be served hot or çold.

PRUNE SOUP

225 g / 8 oz stoned prunes, soaked overnight in
    1.2 litres / 2 pints cold water
1 stick cinnamon
50 g / 2 oz raisins
thinly pared rind of ½ orange
thinly pared rind of ½ lemon
2 tablespoons fine oatmeal

SERVES 6
Per serving: **Energy** 100 kcal / 425 kJ
               Fat negligible
               Fibre 7 g

Put the prunes and the soaking liquid into a saucepan. Add the cinnamon stick, raisins and rinds. Bring to the boil and simmer for about 15 minutes until tender. Discard the cinnamon stick. Purée the mixture in a blender until smooth. Return to the sauce-pan. Stir in the oatmeal and bring to the boil. Simmer for 15–20 minutes, stirring frequently.

JERUSALEM ARTICHOKE SOUP

1 tablespoon olive oil
1 medium onion, chopped
1 garlic clove, chopped
1 large carrot, scrubbed and chopped
750 g / 1½ lb Jerusalem artichokes, scrubbed and
    chopped
1 medium potato, peeled and chopped
600 ml / 1 pint chicken stock
1 sprig parsley
1 bay leaf
freshly ground black pepper

600 ml / 1 pint skimmed milk
½ teaspoon grated nutmeg
TO GARNISH
chopped fresh parsley
wholemeal croûtons

SERVES 4
Per serving: Energy 145 kcal/600 kJ
              Fat   4 g
              Fibre 1 g

Heat the oil in a large saucepan, add the onion and fry until transparent. Add the garlic and carrot and cook for 2–3 minutes longer. Add the artichokes and potato, cover with the stock and bring to the boil. Add the parsley, bay leaf and pepper. Cover and simmer for 20 minutes.

Remove the bay leaf. Purée the soup in a blender with the milk and return it to the rinsed pan. Stir in the nutmeg. Reheat gently. Taste and adjust the seasoning.

Serve very hot, garnished with a little parsley, and with wholemeal croûtons or crusty, warm wholemeal bread.

RED BEAN CHOWDER

100 g / 4 oz red kidney beans, soaked in water
    overnight, or 1 × 425 g (15 oz) can red
    kidney beans and 300 ml / ½ pint beef stock
120 g / 4½ oz lean ground beef
1 large onion, finely chopped
1 × 425 g (15 oz) can tomatoes
1 teaspoon tomato purée
450 ml / ¾ pint beef stock

freshly ground black pepper
about 1 teaspoon chilli powder
1 teaspoon cornflour

SERVES 4
Per serving: Energy 130 kcal/535 kJ
              Fat   2 g
              Fibre 7 g

Chilli powder is very hot and varies in strength according to the brand used, so use it cautiously.

If using dried beans, drain and place in a saucepan with enough water to cover. Bring to the boil, then boil for 10 minutes. Cover and simmer for 1½ hours. Drain and reserve 300 ml / ½ pint of the cooking liquid.

Cook the beef in a pan over a gentle heat with no extra fat for 5 minutes, stirring occasionally. Add the onion and continue cooking for a further 5 minutes. Add the tomatoes, tomato purée, stock, pepper, chilli powder and the drained beans with the reserved liquid. If using canned beans, drain and rinse under cold running water and add with the extra beef stock. Bring to the boil, cover and simmer gently for about 1 hour.

Take off the heat, taste and adjust the seasoning, add the cornflour blended in a little cold water and return the soup to the heat to bring back to the boil. Serve in bowls with hot wholemeal rolls.

OPPOSITE: LENTIL AND HERB SOUP

LENTIL AND HERB SOUP

100 g / 4 oz lentils, red or brown, soaked for 1
   hour in cold water
1.2 litres / 2 pints stock: veal, chicken or game
2 teaspoons olive oil
1 small onion, chopped
1 garlic clove, crushed
100 g / 4 oz spinach beet, or spinach, sliced
freshly ground black pepper
50 g / 2 oz chopped mixed herbs: sorrel, parsley,

chervil, tarragon, lovage and lemon thyme
1 tablespoon lemon juice
150 ml / ¼ pint plain unsweetened yogurt or
   buttermilk

SERVES 4

Per serving:	Energy	105 kcal / 445 kJ
	Fat	2 g
	Fibre	5 g

Drain the lentils and put in a large pan with the stock. Bring to the boil and simmer until they are soft – about 30 minutes for red lentils, and 45 minutes for brown.

Heat the oil in a pan and cook the onion until soft and golden, adding the garlic halfway through. Add the spinach to the lentils when they are soft, with pepper to taste. Simmer until the spinach is cooked,

about 8 minutes, then add the onion, garlic and roughly chopped herbs. Simmer for a further 2–3 minutes, then cool slightly. Purée in a blender and add the lemon juice and yogurt or buttermilk. Serve immediately, or, if it is necessary to reheat, do so very carefully in a double saucepan without allowing the soup to boil. This soup is also good served cold.

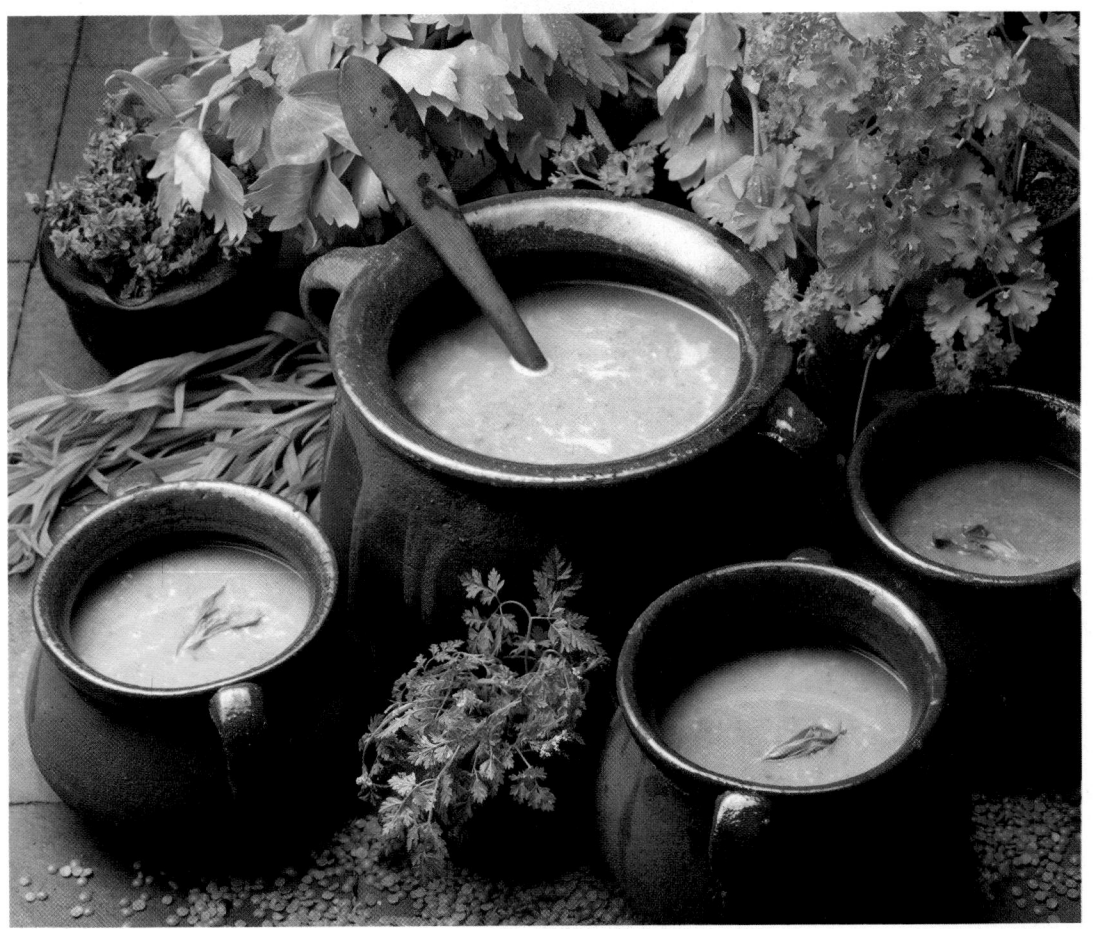

ORANGE BEETROOT SOUP

375 g/13 oz beetroot, peeled and coarsely grated
600 ml/1 pint beef stock
300 ml/½ pint tomato juice, preferably
homemade and unseasoned
300 ml/½ pint unsweetened orange juice
freshly ground black pepper

TO GARNISH
finely chopped chives

SERVES 4
Per serving: **Energy**   60 kcal/260 kJ
                 Fat   negligible
                 Fibre   3 g

Put the beetroot in a saucepan with the stock, bring to the boil and simmer for 30 minutes. Add the tomato and orange juices and season to taste with pepper.

The soup may be served hot or cold sprinkled with chives.

COURGETTE SOUP

450 g/1 lb courgettes, unpeeled and thinly sliced
600 ml/1 pint chicken stock
½ teaspoon chopped fresh basil
½ teaspoon chopped fresh thyme
½ teaspoon chopped fresh marjoram
300 ml/½ pint skimmed milk
freshly ground black pepper

SERVES 4
Per serving: **Energy**   45 kcal/180 kJ
                 Fat   negligible
                 Fibre   2 g

Put the courgettes and stock in a saucepan. Bring to the boil and simmer for about 15 minutes until tender. Leave to cool.

Add the herbs and purée in a blender until smooth. Return the mixture to the saucepan. Stir in the milk and season with pepper. Heat the soup gently but do not allow it to boil.

CURRIED LENTIL SOUP

1 tablespoon oil
2 medium onions, finely chopped
2 garlic cloves, crushed
225 g/8 oz red lentils, soaked for 1 hour in cold
water
1 litre/1¾ pints water
1 bay leaf
½ teaspoon ground ginger
½ teaspoon ground turmeric
2 teaspoons curry powder

freshly ground black pepper
lemon juice
TO GARNISH
chopped parsley

SERVES 6
Per serving: **Energy**   170 kcal/720 kJ
                 Fat   3 g
                 Fibre   6 g

Heat the oil in a pan and cook the onions and garlic over a low heat until soft but not coloured. Add the drained lentils, water, bay leaf, ginger, turmeric, curry powder and pepper. Bring to the boil and simmer gently for 45 minutes, stirring occasionally. Sharpen with lemon juice to taste, adjust the seasoning and serve sprinkled with chopped parsley.

OPPOSITE: CURRIED LENTIL SOUP

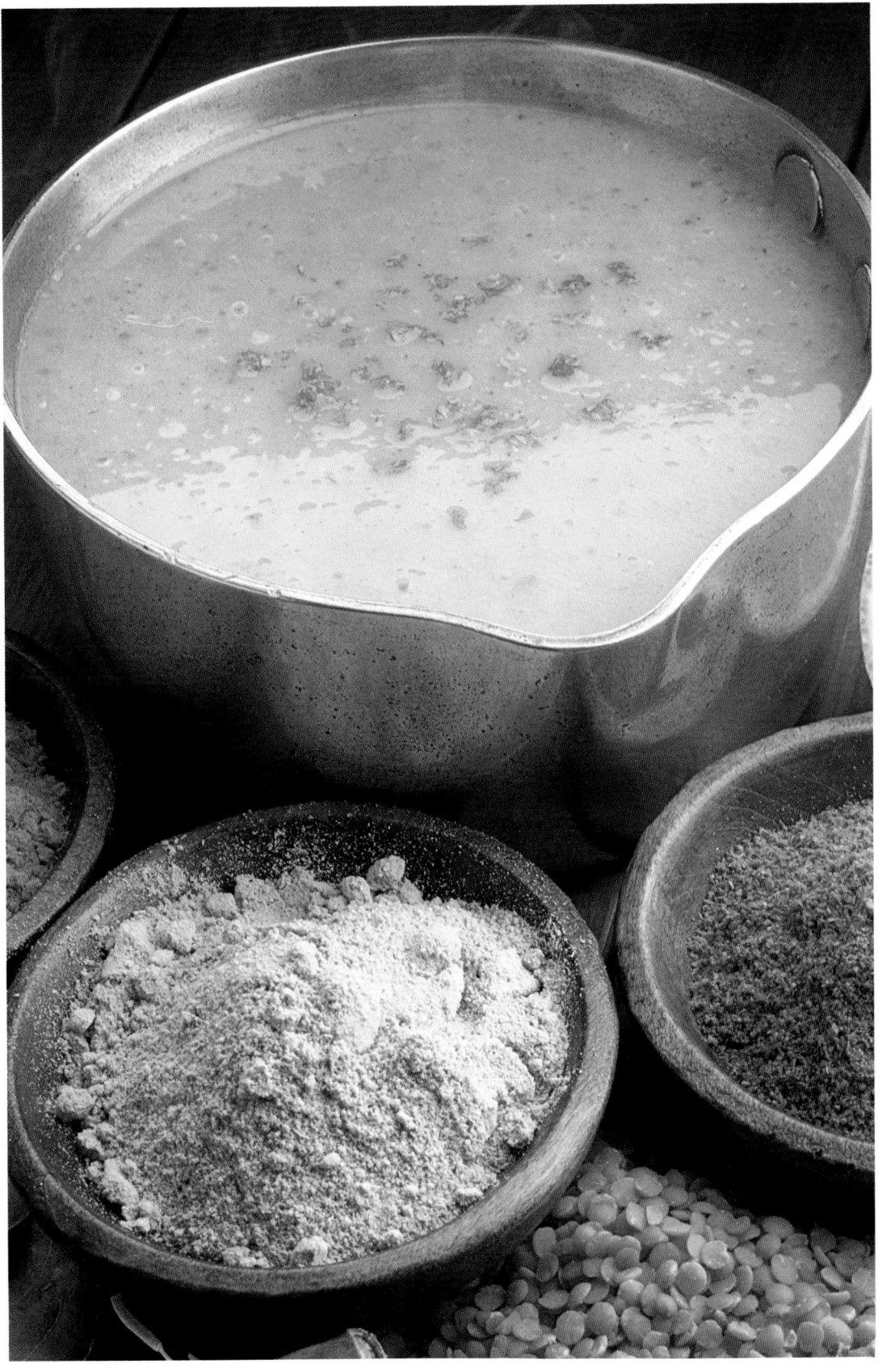

GREEN PEA SOUP

2 × 275 g (10 oz) packets frozen peas,
  preferably petits pois
4 lettuce leaves
900 ml / 1½ pints chicken stock
40 g / 1½ oz green spring onion, diced
freshly ground black pepper

TO GARNISH
chopped mint

SERVES 6
Per serving: **Energy** 50 kcal/220 kJ
                Fat   negligible
                Fibre 7 g

Put all the ingredients in a saucepan, bring to the boil and simmer for 5 minutes. Purée in a blender until smooth.

Serve the soup chilled with chopped fresh mint sprinkled over each portion and with wholemeal rolls.

CARROT AND ORANGE SOUP

1 tablespoon olive oil
1 garlic clove, crushed
1 medium onion, finely chopped
500 g / 1¼ lb carrots, scrubbed and coarsely
  grated
900 ml / 1½ pints water
2 tablespoons orange juice
finely grated zest of 1 orange
1 teaspoon tomato purée
freshly ground black pepper

1 teaspoon cornflour
2 tablespoons cold water
150 ml / ¼ pint skimmed milk
TO GARNISH
1 teaspoon chopped parsley

SERVES 4
Per serving: **Energy** 90 kcal/390 kJ
                Fat   4 g
                Fibre 4 g

Heat the oil in a saucepan, add the garlic, onion and carrots. Stir and cook, covered, for 5 minutes over a low heat. Add the water, orange juice and zest and tomato purée. Season to taste. Simmer, covered, for 30 minutes. Remove from the heat and pour into a blender.

Moisten the cornflour with the cold water and stir into the soup. Stir in the milk and chill in a refrigerator. Before serving, taste and adjust the seasoning and sprinkle with the chopped parsley.

CAULIFLOWER SOUP

200 g / 7 oz cauliflower florets
400 ml / 14 fl oz plain unsweetened yogurt
6 tablespoons chicken stock
75 g / 3 oz red pepper, cored, seeded and chopped
50 g / 2 oz walnuts, chopped
freshly ground black pepper

SERVES 6
Per serving: **Energy** 85 kcal/355 kJ
                Fat   5 g
                Fibre 1 g

Purée all the ingredients in a blender until smooth. Serve chilled with crusty wholemeal rolls.

CUCUMBER AND YOGURT SOUP

1 medium cucumber, washed
600 ml / 1 pint plain unsweetened yogurt
1 garlic clove, crushed
2 teaspoons chopped fresh mint
freshly ground black pepper
TO GARNISH
50 g / 2 oz walnuts, chopped

SERVES 4

Per serving:	Energy	150 kcal/620 kJ
	Fat	8 g
	Fibre	1 g

Leaving the cucumber unpeeled, dice it and put it in a blender with the yogurt, garlic and mint. Blend until smooth. Season with pepper. Serve the soup cold, garnished with chopped walnuts, with crusty wholemeal rolls.

CHILLED AVOCADO SOUP

3 ripe avocados
3–4 tablespoons lemon juice
1 × 425 g (15 oz) can consommé
175 ml / 6 fl oz plain unsweetened yogurt
freshly ground black pepper
TO GARNISH
chopped chives

SERVES 4–6
4 servings

Per serving:	Energy	190 kcal/800 kJ
	Fat	19 g
	Fibre	2 g

6 servings

Per serving:	Energy	125 kcal/530 kJ
	Fat	13 g
	Fibre	2 g

Halve the avocados and scoop out the flesh. Put all the ingredients (except the chives) in a blender and purée at high speed until the mixture is smooth. Sprinkle with a few chopped chives before serving chilled with crusty wholemeal rolls.

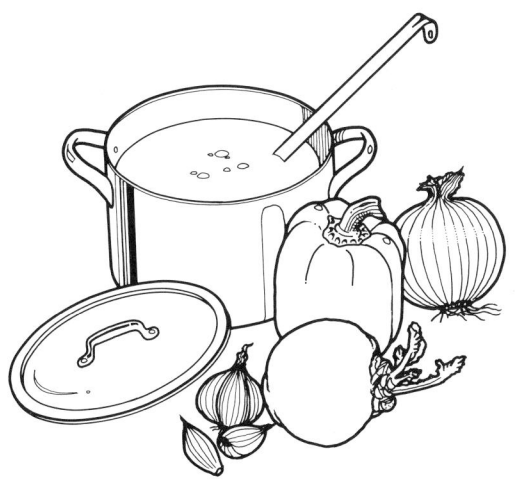

Main Course Dishes

TURKEY-STUFFED PEPPERS

4 large peppers, red, green or yellow mixed
1 tablespoon olive oil
50 g/2 oz lean bacon rashers, rinded and
   chopped
1 onion, finely chopped
50 g/2 oz mushrooms, chopped
250 g/9 oz cooked turkey meat, diced
100 g/4 oz cooked brown rice
1 tablespoon chopped parsley

freshly ground black pepper
25 g/1 oz Edam cheese, grated

SERVES 4
Per serving: **Energy** 305 kcal/1280 kJ
              Fat   9 g
              Fibre 3 g

Cut the tops off the peppers and scoop out the seeds. Blanch the peppers and tops in boiling water for 5 minutes. Rinse in cold water and drain thoroughly.

Heat the oil in a pan. Add the bacon, onion and mushrooms and cook until golden. Stir in the turkey, rice, parsley, and pepper to taste.

Fill the peppers with the turkey mixture and stand them upright in an ovenproof dish. Sprinkle with the grated cheese, replace the tops and cover with foil.

Cook in a preheated moderate oven (180°C, 350°F, Gas Mark 4) for 15 minutes. Remove the foil and cook for a further 10 minutes or until the peppers are tender. Serve hot or cold.

BRAISED PIGEONS

4 young, oven-ready wood pigeons
freshly ground black pepper
2 tablespoons olive oil
1 large onion, chopped
6 rashers lean bacon, rinded, lightly grilled and
   diced
4 tablespoons dry white vermouth or wine
300 ml/½ pint chicken stock

450 g/1 lb shelled fresh peas
1 teaspoon sugar

SERVES 4
Per serving: **Energy** 425 kcal/1775 kJ
              Fat   19 g
              Fibre 6 g

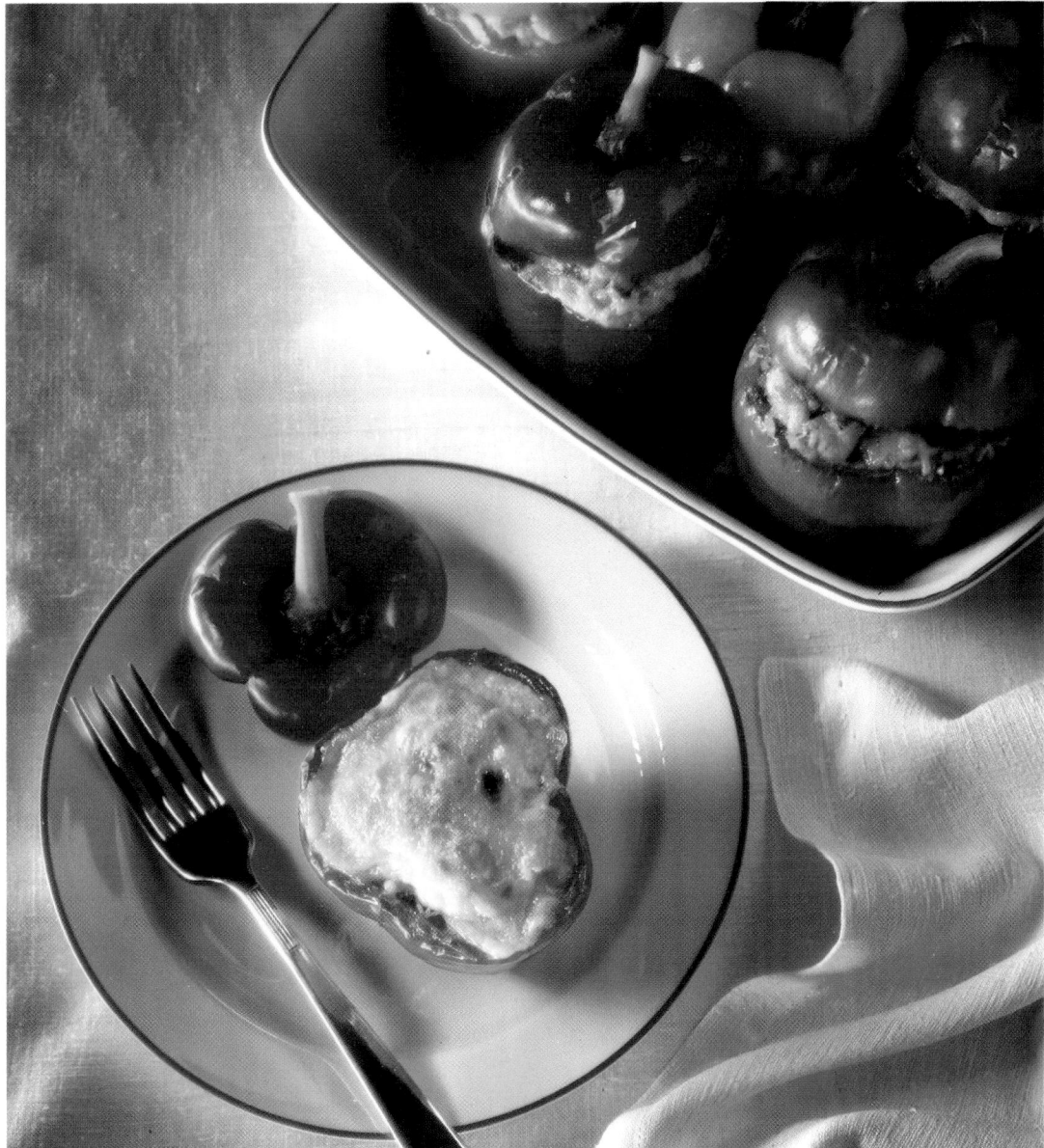

TURKEY–STUFFED PEPPERS

Pigeons tend to be rather dry birds so braising is one of the best ways of cooking them.

Wash the pigeons under running cold water, drain and pat dry with absorbent kitchen paper. Season them inside and out with pepper and tie their legs together.

Heat the oil in a large, flameproof casserole and cook the onion gently for 5 minutes. Increase the heat, add the pigeons and cook, turning as necessary, until golden brown on all sides. Add the bacon, vermouth or wine and the stock, bring to simmering point, cover the casserole tightly and simmer very gently for 1–1½ hours or until the pigeons are almost tender. Check the liquid in the pan occasionally, adding more stock if necessary.

Add the peas and sugar, cover and continue simmering for 20–25 minutes or until the peas and the pigeons are tender. Taste and adjust the seasoning and serve from the casserole.

BRAISED PHEASANT

2 tablespoons olive oil
1 onion, finely chopped
2 celery sticks, thinly sliced
1.25 kg/2½ lb white cabbage, coarsely shredded
6 tablespoons stock, water or dry white wine
8 juniper berries, crushed (optional)
freshly ground black pepper
2 oven-ready pheasants
4 rashers lean bacon, rinded

SERVES 6–8
6 servings
Per serving:	Energy	315 kcal/1325 kJ
	Fat	11 g
	Fibre	7 g

8 servings
Per serving:	Energy	235 kcal/995 kJ
	Fat	8 g
	Fibre	5 g

Braising is an excellent method of cooking either young pheasants, or older birds of indeterminate age. The juices permeate the vegetables with their rich flavour and the birds remain beautifully moist.

Heat the oil in a large, flameproof casserole and cook the onion and celery gently for a few minutes. Add the cabbage, stir to mix thoroughly with the oil and cook gently for 5 minutes, stirring often. Add the stock, water or dry white wine, the juniper berries, if used, and pepper to taste. Continue to cook gently while preparing the pheasants.

Wash the pheasants under running cold water, drain and pat dry with absorbent kitchen paper. Sprinkle inside and out with pepper and tie the legs together. Stretch the bacon rashers out thinly with the blade of a knife and tie them over the breasts of the pheasants with fine string. Put the pheasants in the casserole, moving the cabbage aside so that it surrounds and covers them. Cover the casserole tightly, cook in a preheated moderate oven (160°C, 325°F, Gas Mark 3) for 1–1½ hours.

Arrange a bed of braised cabbage on a hot serving dish and lay the whole, or carved, pheasants on top.

STUFFED CABBAGE LEAVES

12 medium cabbage leaves
1 tablespoon olive oil
1 medium onion, chopped
1 garlic clove, crushed
50 g/2 oz mushrooms, sliced
25 g/1 oz walnuts, chopped
175 g/6 oz cooked brown rice
225 g/8 oz cooked chicken meat, chopped
1 tablespoon tomato purée
2 teaspoons chopped parsley
½ teaspoon dried thyme

freshly ground black pepper
250 ml/8 fl oz chicken stock

SERVES 4–6
4 servings
Per serving:	Energy	275 kcal/1145 kJ
	Fat	12 g
	Fibre	3 g

6 servings
Per serving:	Energy	180 kcal/765 kJ
	Fat	8 g
	Fibre	2 g

Blanch the cabbage leaves in boiling water for 2 minutes. Drain and rinse.

Heat the oil in a frying pan. Add the onion and garlic and cook until softened. Stir in the mushrooms and walnuts and cook for a further 3 minutes. Remove from the heat and add the rice, chicken, tomato purée, herbs and pepper to taste. Mix well.

Divide the chicken mixture between the cabbage leaves and fold them into square parcels. Arrange in a lightly oiled ovenproof dish. Pour over the stock. Cover and cook in a preheated moderate oven (180°C, 350°F, Gas Mark 4) for 30 minutes.

SPINACH AND CHICKEN MOULD

225 g/8 oz young spinach leaves
600 ml/1 pint water
freshly ground black pepper
FILLING
2 tablespoons olive oil
1 medium onion, finely chopped
100 g/4 oz button mushrooms, thinly sliced
2 teaspoons chopped fresh or 1 teaspoon dried
   oregano or marjoram
225 g/8 oz cooked chicken, finely chopped
3 medium tomatoes, diced
¼ medium cucumber, diced
75 g/3 oz Edam cheese, grated
75 g/3 oz fresh wholemeal breadcrumbs

4 tablespoons plain unsweetened yogurt
TO GARNISH
cucumber slices

SERVES 4–6
4 servings
Per serving:	**Energy**	245 kcal/1025 kJ
	Fat	9 g
	Fibre	7 g

6 servings
Per serving:	**Energy**	165 kcal/685 kJ
	Fat	6 g
	Fibre	5 g

Wash the spinach leaves in plenty of cold water and drain. Pour the water into a saucepan, season very lightly and bring to the boil. Put in the spinach leaves and cook for 1–2 minutes only, until just softened. Drain very thoroughly, then line a 23 cm (9 inch) sandwich tin or flan dish with the leaves: leave sufficient hanging over the edges to cover the filling.

Heat the oil in a pan and cook the onion, mushrooms and herbs together until the vegetables are soft. Season well and allow to cool.

Combine all the ingredients, except the spinach leaves, with the yogurt. Spoon into the tin or dish and cover with the spinach leaves. Chill for several hours, then turn out on to a serving plate and garnish with the cucumber slices. Serve the mould cut into slices like a cake.

CHICKEN AND BARLEY CASSEROLE

2 tablespoons olive oil
1 large onion, very finely chopped
225 g/8 oz pearl barley
225 g/8 oz firm button mushrooms, sliced
750 ml/1¼ pints hot chicken stock
½ teaspoon powdered rosemary or 1 sprig fresh
   rosemary
freshly ground black pepper

225 g/8 oz cold cooked chicken, diced
TO GARNISH
chopped parsley

SERVES 4
Per serving:	**Energy**	365 kcal/1540 kJ
	Fat	12 g
	Fibre	5 g

Heat the oil in a large pan. Add the onion, stir over a low heat, then cover and allow to sweat. Add the barley and mushrooms to the onions. Toss to coat well with the oil, then cook for 3–4 minutes. Pour in the stock and rosemary (leave the sprig whole and remove before serving) and add pepper to taste. Mix in the chicken. Transfer to a casserole. Cover and bake in a preheated moderate oven (180°C, 350°F, Gas Mark 4) for about 1 hour until the barley is tender. Sprinkle with the parsley.

CURRIED CHICKEN WITH AVOCADOS

450 g / 1 lb long-grain brown rice
1 tablespoon olive oil
1 medium onion, finely chopped
2 teaspoons curry powder
1 teaspoon tomato purée
150 ml / ¼ pint dry red wine
150 ml / ¼ pint chicken stock
1 bay leaf
freshly ground black pepper
450 ml / ¾ pint plain unsweetened yogurt
100 g / 4 oz frozen sweetcorn kernels, cooked
tablespoon chopped parsley
450 g / 1 lb cooked chicken meat
2 ripe avocados
3 tablespoons lemon juice
TO GARNISH
mustard and cress
parsley sprig
cayenne pepper

SERVES 6
Per serving: Energy 545 kcal / 2300 kJ
Fat 17 g
Fibre 5 g

Cook the rice in boiling water for about 15 minutes or until tender.

Meanwhile heat the oil in another saucepan. Add the onion and fry until softened. Stir in the curry powder and cook for a further 2 minutes. Add the tomato purée, red wine, stock, bay leaf and pepper to taste and bring to the boil, stirring well. Simmer for 10 minutes.

Remove the pan from the heat and cool. Discard the bay leaf, then stir in the yogurt. Liquidize the sauce in a blender for a smooth texture.

Drain the rice and cool.

Mix the rice with the corn and parsley and pile in a ring around the edge of a serving platter. Place the chicken in the centre and pour over some of the curry sauce. Peel, stone and slice the avocados and coat with lemon juice to prevent discoloration. Arrange around the chicken. Chill lightly before serving garnished with mustard and cress, parsley and cayenne pepper. Serve the sauce separately.

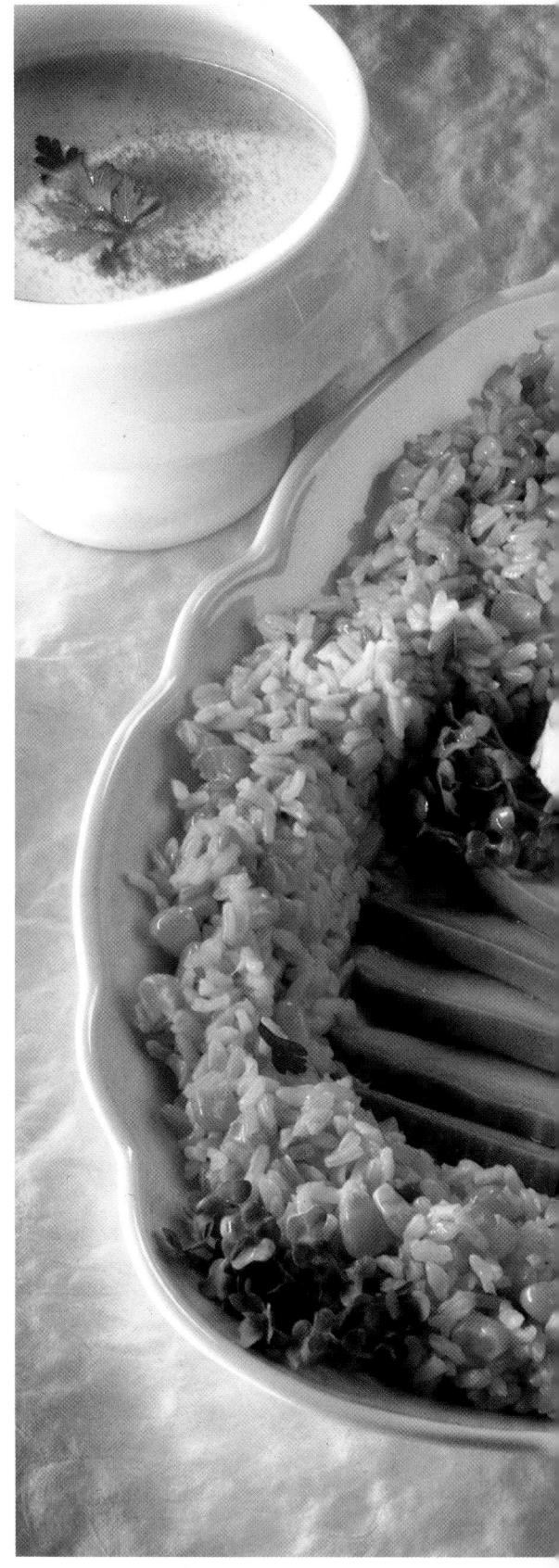

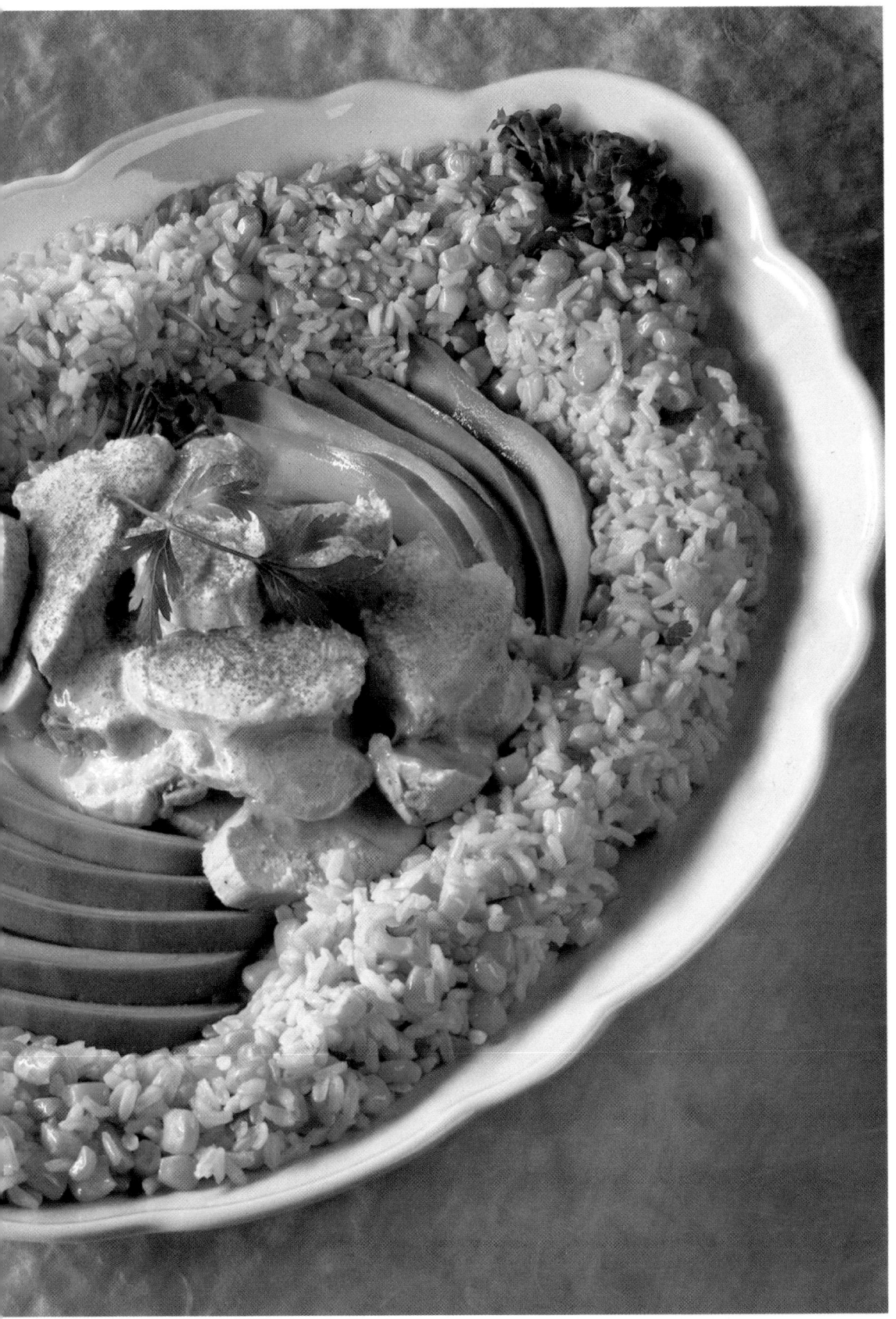

STEAMED BACON AND CARROT PUDDING

175 g/6 oz self-raising wholemeal flour
50 g/2 oz margarine
4 lean bacon rashers, rinded and diced
1 tablespoon chopped parsley
225 g/8 oz carrots, scrubbed and grated
2 onions, finely chopped
1 teaspoon caster sugar
½ teaspoon dried thyme

freshly ground black pepper
120 ml/4 fl oz chicken stock
2 eggs, beaten

SERVES 4

Per serving:	Energy	325 kcal/1375 kJ
	Fat	14 g
	Fibre	8 g

Sift the flour into a bowl. Rub in the margarine until the mixture resembles crumbs. Add the bacon, parsley, carrots, onions, sugar, thyme and pepper to taste and mix well. Stir in the stock and eggs.

Pour into a lightly oiled 1.2 litre (2 pint) pudding basin. Cover and steam for 2 hours. Serve hot.

BAKED TROUT

2 tablespoons olive oil
2 garlic cloves, crushed
2 onions, finely chopped
100 g/4 oz mushrooms, chopped
2 tablespoons capers
2 tablespoons wholemeal flour
25 g/1 oz ground almonds
4 × 225 g (8 oz) trout, cleaned, washed and
    dried
2 tablespoons chopped parsley

pinch of chopped marjoram
½ teaspoon freshly ground black pepper
150 ml/¼ pint chicken stock
TO GARNISH
toasted flaked almonds

SERVES 4

Per serving:	Energy	370 kcal/1560 kJ
	Fat	20 g
	Fibre	4 g

Heat the oil in a large, shallow flameproof casserole or heavy-based pan. Add the garlic and onions and cook gently for 5 minutes until the onions are soft and golden, stirring occasionally. Stir in the mushrooms, capers, flour and ground almonds and cook this mixture gently for a further 3 minutes.

Put the trout on top of the onion mixture, then sprinkle with the parsley, marjoram and pepper. Pour on the stock.

Bake in a preheated moderately hot oven (200°C, 400°F, Gas Mark 6) for 25 minutes, basting twice. Sprinkle the trout with the toasted almonds and serve immediately.

LEMON MACKEREL

50 g/2 oz fresh wholemeal breadcrumbs
grated rind of 1 lemon
1 teaspoon chopped parsley
½ teaspoon dried mixed herbs
2 tablespoons skimmed milk
freshly ground black pepper

4 mackerel, cleaned
2 tablespoons lemon juice

SERVES 4

Per serving:	Energy	200 kcal/830 kJ
	Fat	13 g
	Fibre	1 g

Mix together the breadcrumbs, lemon rind, herbs, milk and pepper to taste. Stuff the fish with this mixture, then close the openings with wooden cocktail sticks.

Arrange the fish in an ovenproof dish, in one layer, and sprinkle over the lemon juice. Cover and cook in a preheated moderate oven (180°C, 350°F, Gas Mark 4) for 35–40 minutes or until the fish flakes easily when tested with a fork.

VARIATION
Replace the lemon with an orange and the dried mixed herbs with dried thyme.

SPICED FISH CASSEROLE

3 large tomatoes, sliced
2 celery sticks, finely chopped
1 garlic clove, crushed
50 g/2 oz mushrooms, sliced
freshly ground black pepper
pinch of grated nutmeg
1 teaspoon chopped parsley
1 teaspoon chopped basil
1 bay leaf
1 onion, sliced

1 carrot, scrubbed and sliced
750 g/1½ lb cod fillets
3 tablespoons wine vinegar
150 ml/¼ pint water

SERVES 4
Per serving: **Energy** 165 kcal/685 kJ
              Fat 1 g
              Fibre 2 g

Arrange half the tomato slices in an ovenproof dish and cover with the celery, garlic and mushrooms. Season well with pepper, then sprinkle with the nutmeg and parsley. Add the basil and the bay leaf and top with the onion and carrot.

Arrange the fish on top of this mixture, then cover with the remaining tomato slices. Pour on the vinegar and water. Cover and bake in a preheated moderate oven (180°C, 350°F, Gas Mark 4) for 40 minutes. Serve hot.

FISHERMEN'S MUSSELS

48 mussels
6 shallots, chopped
300 ml/½ pint dry cider
50 g/2 oz rolled oats
2 tablespoons chopped parsley
freshly ground black pepper

SERVES 4
Per serving: **Energy** 160 kcal/660 kJ
              Fat 3 g
              Fibre 2 g

Wash the mussels and scrub them very thoroughly. Discard any which are open. Put them in a heavy pan with the shallots and cider. Cover and cook over high heat for 5 minutes until all the mussels have opened; discard any which are still closed.

Reserving the cooking liquid, lift out the mussels and discard the top shell from each one. Divide them equally between four individual soup bowls and keep hot.

Put the oats in a saucepan and stir in the cooking liquid gradually. Bring to the boil slowly and simmer until the sauce has thickened slightly, stirring constantly. Stir in the parsley, then add pepper to taste. Pour the sauce over the mussels and serve immediately.

BAKED APPLE MACKEREL

4 fresh mackerel fillets
2 teaspoons made mustard
freshly ground black pepper
450 g / 1 lb potatoes, peeled and thinly sliced
1 medium onion, thinly sliced
1 teaspoon finely chopped fresh sage, or savory
    or parsley
1 large cooking apple, peeled and thinly sliced

150 ml / ¼ pint dry cider
boiling water

SERVES 4
Per serving: **Energy** 535 kcal / 2255 kJ
                Fat   33 g
                Fibre   3 g

Trim the fish fillets neatly and spread with the mustard. Season with pepper and roll up. Oil an ovenproof dish lightly and cover the bottom with half the sliced potatoes. Scatter over the onion slices and season with pepper and chosen herb. Cover the potatoes and onions with the apple slices and place the mackerel rolls on top. Arrange the remaining potatoes over the fish and season with more pepper. Add the cider and enough boiling water to half fill the dish.

Cover with foil and bake in a preheated moderate oven (180°C, 350°F, Gas Mark 4) for 45 minutes. Remove the foil and continue baking for 30 minutes or until the potatoes are golden brown. Serve this dish very hot.

VARIATION
Use fresh herrings or pilchards instead of mackerel. All are fatty fish, but their fat content varies according to the time of year, being lowest in the winter months.

SKATE WITH COURGETTES

4 × 225 g (8 oz) pieces skate
3 tablespoons lemon juice
freshly ground black pepper
1 tablespoon olive oil
1 small onion, thinly sliced
4 small courgettes, cut into sticks
100 g / 4 oz frozen peas
50 g / 2 oz anchovies, wiped and chopped

1 tablespoon capers
TO GARNISH
lemon wedges

SERVES 4
Per serving: **Energy** 300 kcal / 1255 kJ
                Fat   11 g
                Fibre   4 g

Line a shallow ovenproof dish with lightly oiled foil, place the fish on top and sprinkle with the lemon juice, and pepper to taste. Cover with more foil and cook in a preeated moderately hot oven (200°C, 400°F, Gas Mark 6) for 20 minutes. Place on a warmed serving dish and keep warm. Reserve the cooking liquor.

Heat the oil in a small pan, add the onion and cook until soft but not browned.
Add the courgettes and peas and cook gently for a further 5 minutes. Add the anchovies, capers, pepper to taste and the reserved liquor and heat gently. Spoon over the fish and garnish the dish with lemon wedges.

OPPOSITE: SKATE WITH COURGETTES

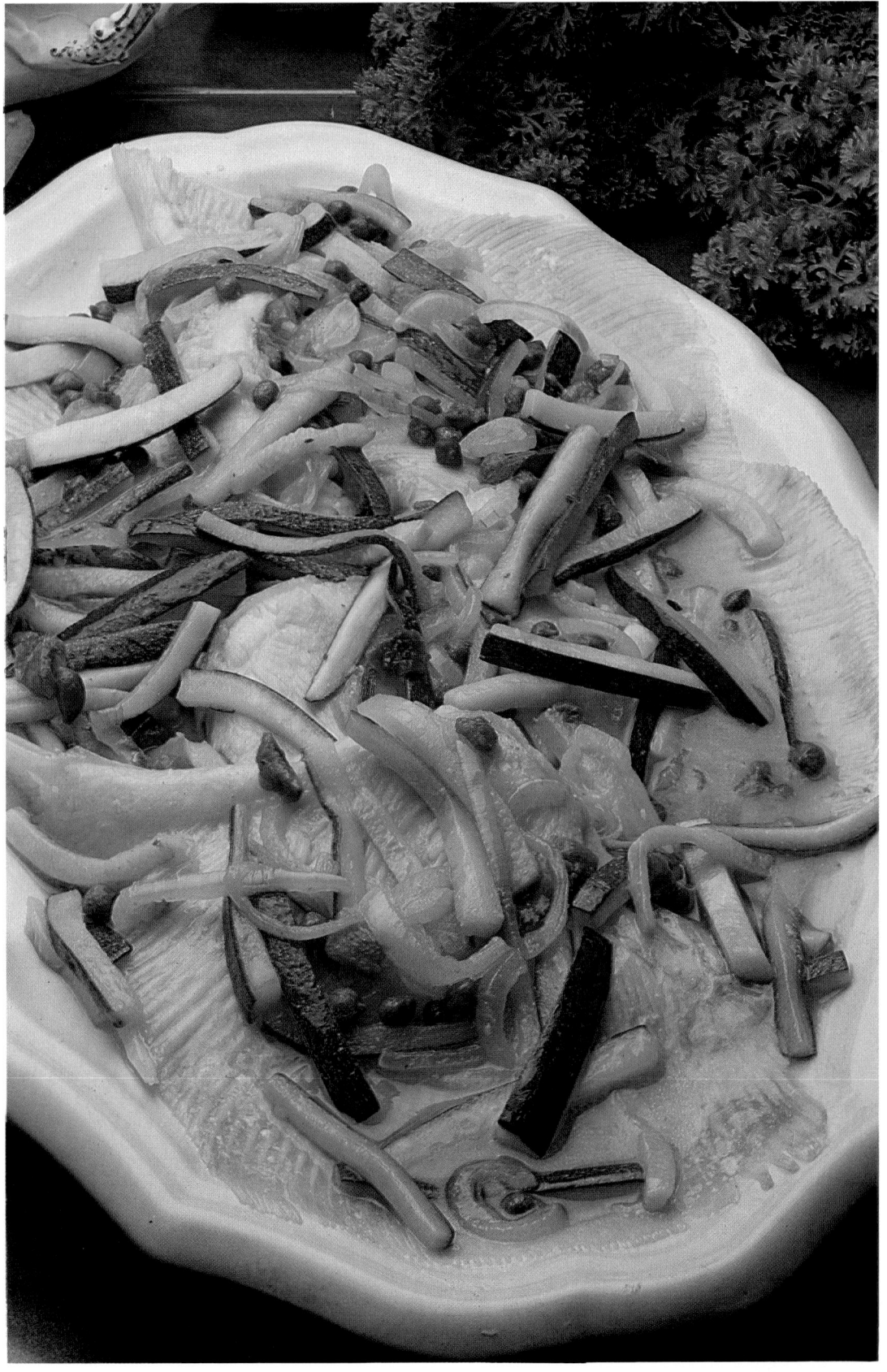

STUFFED GRAPEFRUIT

2 large grapefruit, halved
225 g/8 oz white fish (e.g. cod or haddock), cut
*   into 1 cm/½ inch cubes*
40 g/1½ oz walnuts, chopped
40 g/1½ oz red pepper, cored, seeded and diced
½ teaspoon ground ginger

SERVES 4
Per serving: Energy 110 kcal/455 kJ
**   Fat**   6 g
**   Fibre** 1 g

Use a grapefruit knife to scoop out the segments carefully. Setting the skins aside, mix the fruit with the remaining ingredients. Divide the mixture between the reserved grapefruit skins. Cover lightly with foil and cook in a preheated moderate oven (180°C, 350°F, Gas Mark 4) for 15 minutes.

BROCCOLI WITH YOGURT SAUCE

500 g/1¼ lb broccoli
300 ml/½ pint plain unsweetened yogurt,
*   stabilized (page 9)*
1 garlic clove, crushed
1 teaspoon dried mint or 3–4 fresh mint leaves,
*   chopped*
freshly ground black pepper

SERVES 4
Per serving: Energy 80 kcal/335 kJ
**   Fat**   4 g
**   Fibre** 5 g

Steam the broccoli under a tightly fitting lid for 12–15 minutes or until tender.

Meanwhile, heat the yogurt, garlic, mint and pepper to taste gently in a small saucepan, stirring until thickened. When the broccoli is cooked, drain and put it into a warmed serving dish. Pour over the yogurt sauce and serve immediately.

LEMON GLAZED CARROTS

350 g/12 oz young carrots, scrubbed and
*   trimmed*
15 g/½ oz margarine
1 teaspoon muscovado sugar
300 ml/½ pint stock
1 tablespoon finely chopped mint
1 tablespoon lemon juice
freshly ground black pepper

SERVES 4
Per serving: Energy 50 kcal/220 kJ
**   Fat**   3 g
**   Fibre** 3 g

Put the carrots into a saucepan with the margarine and sugar. Barely cover with the stock. Bring to the boil and cook, uncovered, over a moderate heat until all the liquid has been absorbed and the carrots are glazed. Stir in the mint and the lemon juice, season with pepper, and simmer for a further 2 minutes.

CELERY WITH ORANGE AND NUTS

1 head celery, cut into 5 cm/2 inch lengths
4 tablespoons orange juice
grated rind 1 orange
1 orange, peeled and segmented
25 g/1 oz sultanas
25 g/1 oz walnuts, halved
freshly ground black pepper

SERVES 4
Per serving: **Energy** 100 kcal/410 kJ
               Fat 3 g
               Fibre 2 g

Mix together all the ingredients in an ovenproof dish, with pepper to taste. Cover and cook in a preheated moderate oven (180°C, 350°F, Gas Mark 4) for 30–40 minutes or until the celery is just tender. Serve this dish hot.

GRILLED COURGETTES WITH MUSTARD

450 g/1 lb courgettes, scrubbed and cut in half
   lengthways
15 g/½ oz margarine, melted
1 tablespoon Dijon mustard

SERVES 4
Per serving: **Energy** 55 kcal/230 kJ
               Fat 4 g
               Fibre 6 g

Brush the courgettes with the melted margarine and place them, cut side down, in a heated grill pan. Grill under a high heat until they are lightly brown. Turn them over and spread with the mustard. Return to the grill and cook until golden.

GREEN PEPPERS AND BEANS

450 g/1 lb green beans
2 green peppers, cored, seeded and chopped
2 medium onions, finely chopped

freshly ground black pepper
dried thyme
40 g/1½ oz margarine

SERVES 4–6
4 servings
Per serving: **Energy** 100 kcal/410 kJ
               Fat 8 g
               Fibre 5 g

6 servings
Per serving: **Energy** 65 kcal/275 kJ
               Fat 6 g
               Fibre 3 g

If the beans are large, cut them in half. Make layers of the vegetables in a lightly oiled casserole, beginning and ending with the beans. Sprinkle each layer with black pepper and a little thyme, and dot with the margarine.

    Cover and cook in a preheated moderate oven (180°C, 350°F, Gas Mark 4) for about 1 hour or until the vegetables are very tender. *Illustrated on p. 32.*

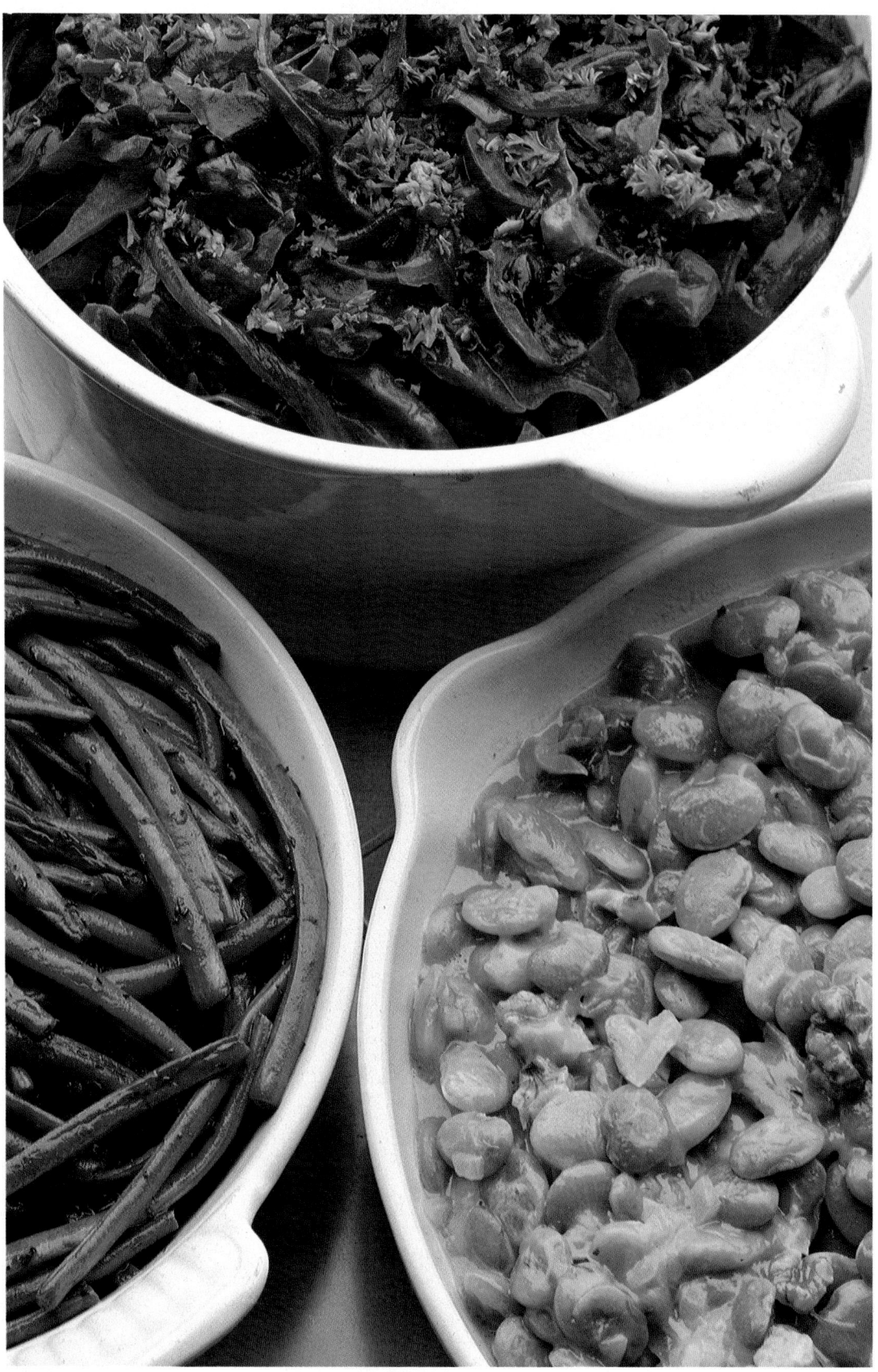

RED CABBAGE WITH APPLE

1 kg/2 lb red cabbage, shredded
1 tablespoon olive oil
1 medium onion, thinly sliced
2 medium dessert apples, cored and sliced
3 tablespoons water
3 tablespoons wine vinegar
4 teaspoons muscovado sugar
freshly ground black pepper
50 g/2 oz rolled oats
TO GARNISH
chopped parsley

SERVES 4–6
4 servings
Per serving: **Energy** 195 kcal/825 kJ
               Fat 5 g
               Fibre 12 g
6 servings
Per serving: **Energy** 130 kcal/550 kJ
               Fat 3 g
               Fibre 8 g

Blanch the cabbage in boiling water for 1 minute, then drain well. Heat the oil in a flameproof casserole and cook the onion gently until soft. Add the apples and cook for a further 5 minutes. Remove the apple mixture from the casserole with a slotted spoon.

Make alternate layers of the cabbage and apple mixture in the casserole, beginning and ending with cabbage. Sprinkle each layer with the water, vinegar, sugar and pepper to taste. Cover tightly and cook in a preheated moderate oven (160°C, 325°F, Gas Mark 3) for 2 hours, stirring occasionally and adding more water if necessary.

Mix the oats with a little of the liquid from the casserole, then stir this into the casserole. Cook gently on top of the cooker until thickened. Serve garnished with parsley.

NUTTY BROAD BEAN CASSEROLE

2 × 300 g (10 oz) packets frozen broad beans,
  thawed
1 tablespoon olive oil
1 medium onion, finely chopped
150 ml/¼ pint chicken stock
100 g/4 oz Edam cheese, grated
1½ teaspoons made mustard
1 teaspoon Worcestershire sauce

freshly ground black pepper
100 g/4 oz walnuts, chopped

SERVES 4
Per serving: **Energy** 320 kcal/1335 kJ
               Fat 22 g
               Fibre 9 g

Cook the beans in boiling water for 5 minutes and drain well.

Heat the oil in a pan and cook the onion gently until soft. Stir in the stock and bring to the boil. Add the cheese, stir until melted, then mix in the mustard, Worcestershire sauce and pepper to taste. Stir in beans and walnuts gently.

Transfer the mixture to a lightly oiled casserole and cook in a preheated moderate oven (180°C, 350°F, Gas Mark 4) for 30 minutes.

OPPOSITE, LEFT: GREEN PEPPERS AND BEANS
(P.31); TOP: RED CABBAGE WITH APPLE;
RIGHT: NUTTY BROAD BEAN CASSEROLE

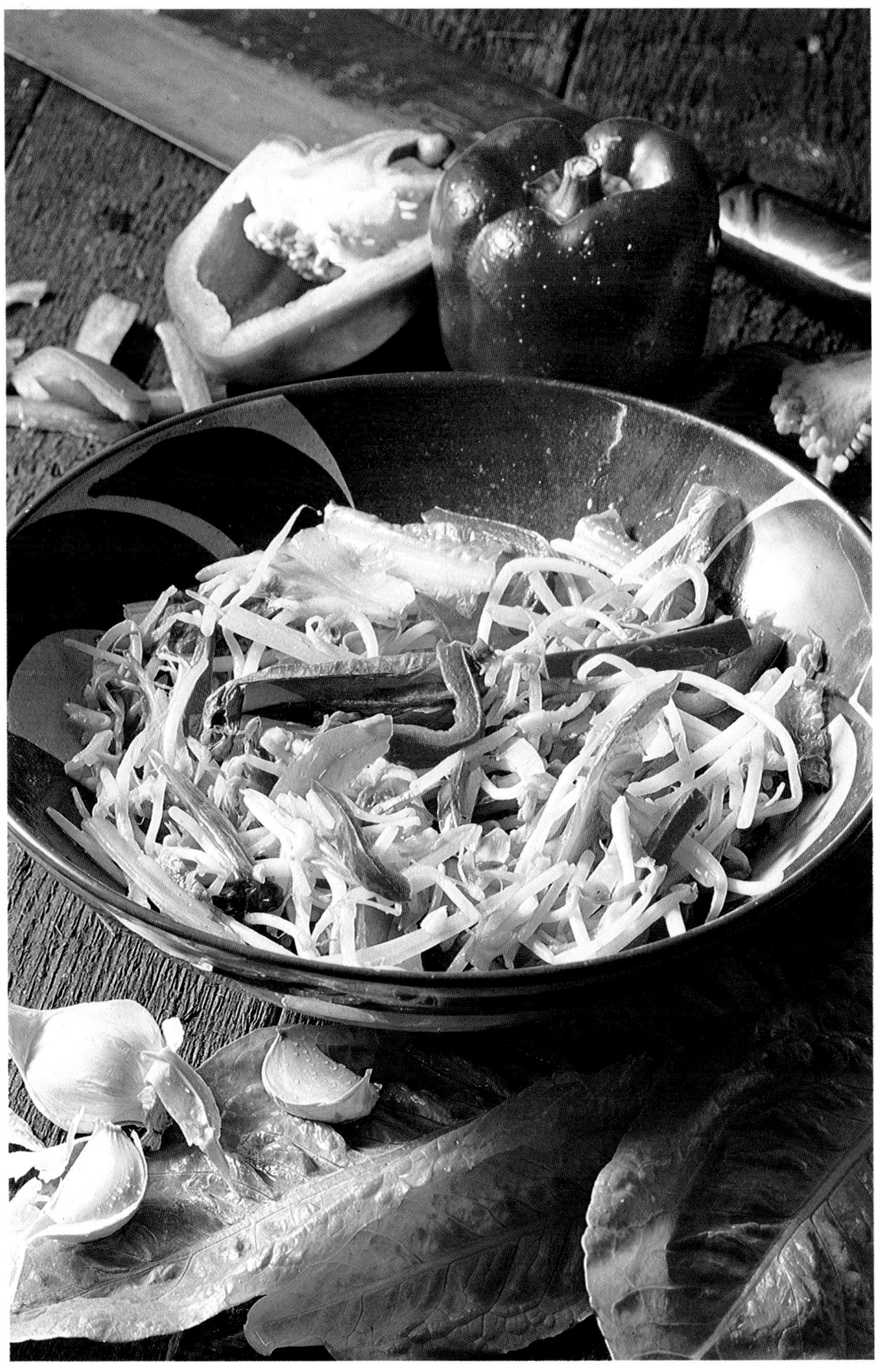

STIR-FRIED MIXED VEGETABLES

2 tablespoons vegetable oil
1 medium onion, thinly sliced
3 garlic cloves, crushed
½ green pepper, cored, seeded and sliced
½ red pepper, cored, seeded and sliced
¼ cucumber, chopped
2 celery sticks, chopped

2 spring onions, chopped
3–4 lettuce leaves, chopped
225 g/8 oz bean-sprouts
1½ teaspoons caster sugar
1 tablespoon soy sauce
2 tablespoons chicken stock

SERVES 3–4

3 servings
Per serving: **Energy** 135 kcal/565 kJ
                 Fat 10 g
                 Fibre 4 g

4 servings
Per serving: **Energy** 100 kcal/425 kJ
                 Fat 5 g
                 Fibre 2 g

Heat the oil in a wok or frying pan, add the onion and garlic and stir-fry for 30 seconds. Add all the other vegetables and toss until well coated.

Sprinkle in the sugar, soy sauce and chicken stock. Stir-fry the mixture gently for 1½ minutes. Transfer to a warmed serving dish and serve hot.

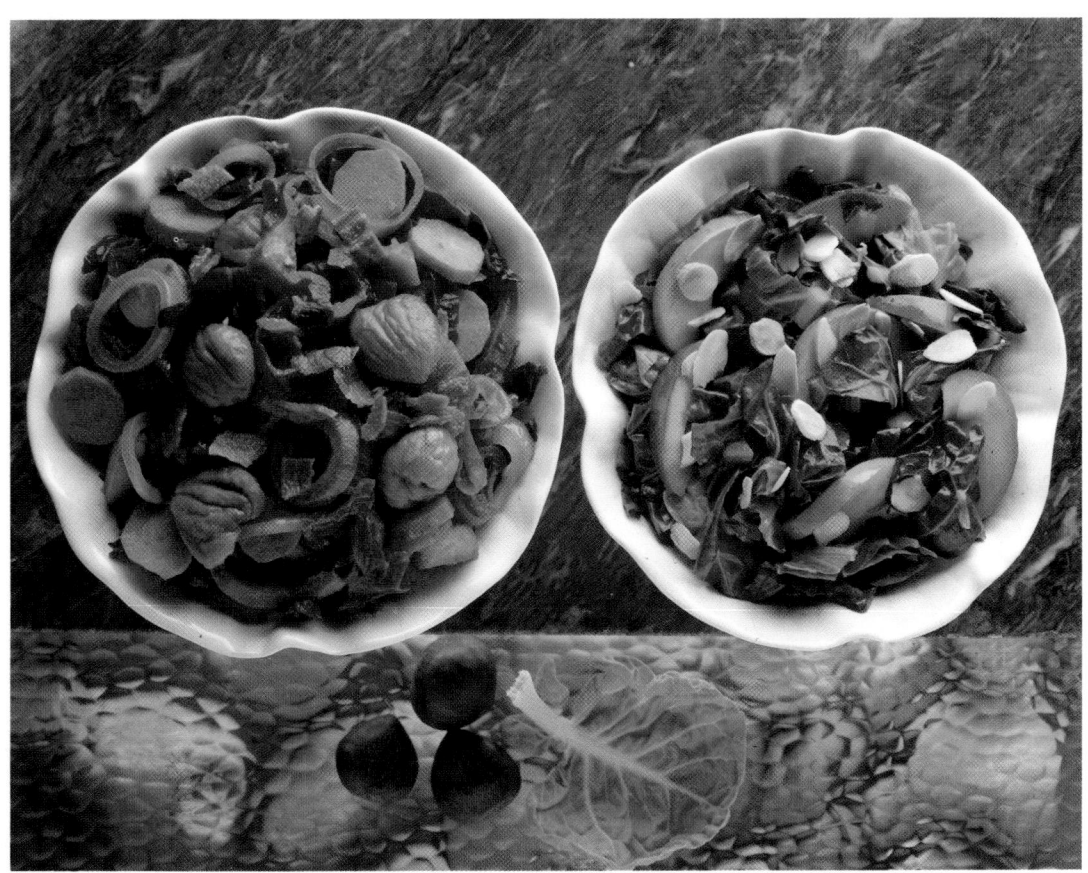

OPPOSITE: STIR-FRIED MIXED VEGETABLES

ABOVE, LEFT: BRAISED RED CABBAGE WITH CHESTNUTS (P. 36); RIGHT: WINTER CABBAGE AND APPLES (P. 36)

BRAISED RED CABBAGE WITH CHESTNUTS

1 tablespoon olive oil
2 large onions, sliced
1 kg / 2 lb red cabbage, trimmed and cut into
    1 cm / ½ inch slices
100 g / 4 oz lean streaky bacon, rinded, lightly
    grilled and chopped
4 carrots, scrubbed and thinly sliced
500 g / 1 lb Bramley or other tart cooking apples,
    peeled, cored and roughly chopped
2 garlic cloves, crushed
pinch of ground cloves
pinch of freshly grated nutmeg
freshly ground black pepper

1 bouquet garni
150 ml / ¼ pint dry red wine
24 whole chestnuts, skinned (see Note, below)

SERVES 4–6
4 servings
Per serving:	Energy	305 kcal / 1290 kJ
	Fat	7 g
	Fibre	18 g

6 servings
Per serving:	Energy	205 kcal / 860 kJ
	Fat	5 g
	Fibre	12 g

This piquant dish is a delicious accompaniment to poultry.

Heat the oil in a pan, add the onions and cook gently for 5 minutes without browning.

Arrange the cabbage, bacon and onions, carrots, apples and garlic, in layers in a deep ovenproof dish, seasoning each layer with cloves, nutmeg and pepper to taste. Put the bouquet garni in the centre of the casserole, then pour over the wine.

Cover and cook in a preheated moderate oven (160°C, 325°F, Gas Mark 3) for 1 hour. Remove from the oven and stir in the chestnuts, cover and return to the oven for a further 1–1½ hours, until the vegetables are tender. Discard the bouquet garni. *Illustrated on p. 35.*

NOTE To skin chestnuts, place a few at a time in a pan of boiling water. Boil for 4 minutes, then drain. Protecting your hand with a glove or cloth, and using a sharp knife, peel off the shell and furry inner skin while the chestnuts are still hot.

WINTER CABBAGE AND APPLES

1 tablespoon olive oil
1 onion, finely chopped
1 small firm white or green cabbage, trimmed
    and cut into 1 cm / ½ inch slices
4 red dessert apples, cored and sliced
finely grated rind of 1 lemon
3 tablespoons lemon juice
2 teaspoons muscovado sugar
freshly ground black pepper
150 ml / ¼ pint well-flavoured chicken stock
TO GARNISH
25 g / 1 oz flaked almonds, lightly toasted

SERVES 4–6
4 servings
Per serving:	Energy	140 kcal / 585 kJ
	Fat	7 g
	Fibre	5 g

6 servings
Per serving:	Energy	90 kcal / 390 kJ
	Fat	5 g
	Fibre	4 g

Heat the oil in a pan, add the onion and cook gently for 5 minutes without browning. Add the cabbage and mix well. Add the apples, lemon rind and juice and the sugar, and season well with pepper. Pour over the stock and bring to the boil, then lower the heat, cover and simmer for 40–45 minutes, stirring occasionally. Serve sprinkled with the toasted almonds. *Illustrated on p. 35.*

SPINACH WITH FLAKED ALMONDS

1 kg/2 lb leaf spinach, spinach beet or orache
1 tablespoon olive oil
½ onion, finely chopped
freshly ground black pepper
grated nutmeg
1 egg yolk
4 tablespoons plain unsweetened yogurt,
  stabilized (page 8)
50 g/2 oz flaked almonds, toasted

SERVES 4
Per serving: **Energy** 200 kcal/850 kJ
               Fat 10 g
               Fibre 18 g

Sort the spinach, place in a sieve, rinse and drain thoroughly. Tear the leaves into manageable pieces. Heat the oil in a large pan, add the onion and cook for 2–3 minutes until softened. Add the spinach, a little at a time, turning it in the oil to coat. Season with pepper and nutmeg to taste. Cook over a low heat for 10–15 minutes, until tender depending upon the thickness of the spinach leaves.

Beat the egg yolk with the yogurt and stir into the spinach mixture. Immediately remove the spinach from the heat and transfer to a warmed serving bowl. Fold the almonds into the spinach and serve immediately.

GRILLED LEEKS

500 g/1¼ lb leeks, scrubbed and cut into 4 cm/
  1½ inch lengths
15 g/½ oz margarine, softened
1 tablespoon grated Parmesan cheese
2 teaspoons Dijon mustard

SERVES 4
Per serving: **Energy** 75 kcal/320 kJ
               Fat 4 g
               Fibre 4 g

Cook the leeks in boiling water for about 10 minutes. Drain and transfer to a shallow flameproof dish. Cream together the margarine, cheese and mustard and spread the mixture over the leeks. Cook under a preheated hot grill until golden.

BRAISED SWEETCORN

2 × 225g (8oz) cans sweetcorn, drained
1 × 225g (8oz) packet frozen peas
2 tablespoons red pepper, diced
50g/2oz lean bacon, rinded, grilled and
  chopped
freshly ground black pepper
175ml/6fl oz chicken stock
2 tablespoons dry white wine

SERVES 4
Per serving: **Energy** 145 kcal/610 kJ
               Fat 3g
               Fibre 10g

Combine the sweetcorn, frozen peas, red pepper and bacon. Season with pepper and put into an ovenproof casserole. Mix together the stock and wine and pour over the vegetables in the casserole.

Cover and bake in a preheated moderate oven (180°C, 350°F, Gas Mark 4) for 20 minutes or until the peas are tender.

BAMBOO SHOOTS WITH BROCCOLI

2–3 tablespoons olive oil
375 g / 13 oz broccoli, divided into florets
½ × 225 g (8 oz) can bamboo shoots, drained
   with juice reserved and cut into thin strips
1 medium onion, finely chopped
pinch of ground cinnamon
cayenne pepper
1 egg yolk

2 tablespoons plain unsweetened yogurt,
   stabilized (page 8)
dash of Tabasco sauce

SERVES 4
Per serving: **Energy** 160 kcal / 670 kJ
           Fat   13 g
           Fibre   4 g

Heat the oil in a frying pan. Add the broccoli, bamboo shoots and onion and fry for 3–4 minutes. Add a little of the reserved bamboo shoot juice, the cinnamon and cayenne pepper to taste, blending well. Simmer, over a low heat, for 2–3 minutes.

Beat the egg yolk with the yogurt and Tabasco sauce. Remove the pan from the heat and when off the boil and cooled slightly, add the egg mixture, blending well. Transfer to a serving dish and serve immediately.

BRAISED FENNEL

2 tablespoons olive oil
3 heads fennel, trimmed and quartered
   lengthways
150 ml / ¼ pint chicken stock
1 tablespoon lemon juice
freshly ground black pepper
1 tablespoon grated Parmesan cheese
1 tablespoon wholemeal breadcrumbs

SERVES 4
Per serving: **Energy** 110 kcal / 470 kJ
           Fat   9 g
           Fibre   1 g

Heat the oil in a large heavy-based pan, add the fennel and cook, stirring carefully until well coated in the oil.

Pour in the stock and lemon juice, adding pepper to taste. Cover and simmer gently for 35–40 minutes. Sprinkle with the cheese and breadcrumbs and place under a preheated hot grill until golden brown. Serve immediately.

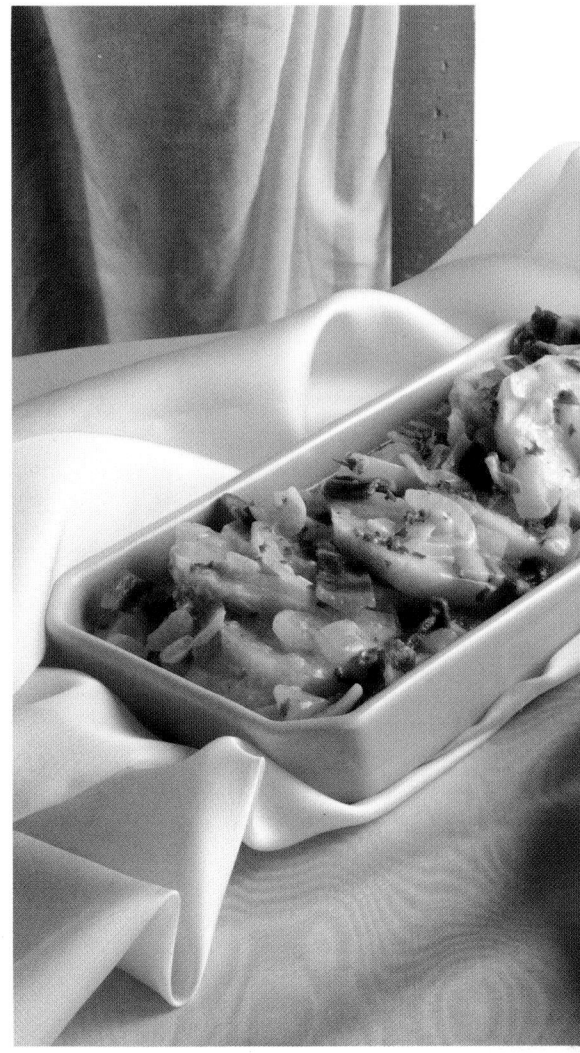

CLOCKWISE FROM TOP: BRAISED FENNEL,
KOHLRABI CASSEROLE (P. 79), BAMBOO
SHOOTS WITH BROCCOLI, CELERY WITH
SWEETCORN

CELERY WITH SWEETCORN

1 tablespoon olive oil
½ head celery, cut into 5 cm / 2 inch lengths
3 tomatoes, chopped
250 ml / 8 fl oz chicken stock
1 × 200 g (7 oz) can sweetcorn kernels, drained
pinch of chilli powder
freshly ground black pepper

1 tablespoon chopped parsley
pinch of cayenne pepper (optional)

SERVES 4
Per serving: **Energy** 120 kcal / 510 kJ
               Fat 8 g
               Fibre 4 g

Heat the oil in a pan. Add the celery and cook over a low heat for 7–8 minutes. Add the tomatoes and stock and cook over a low heat for about 8 minutes. Add the sweetcorn, chilli powder and pepper to taste. Bring to the boil.

Transfer to a warmed serving dish and sprinkle with chopped parsley, and cayenne pepper if liked. Serve immediately.

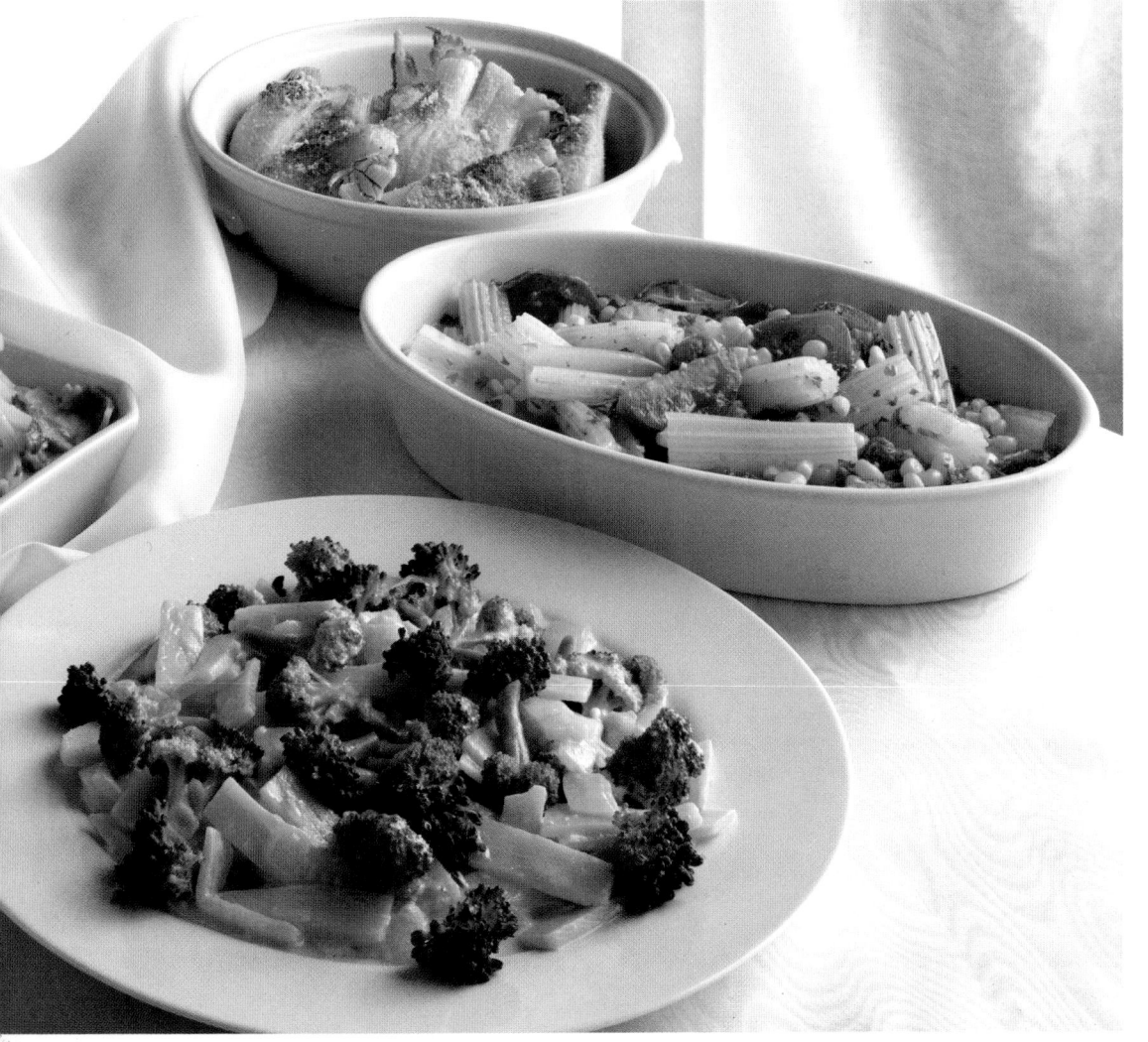

International Dishes

TUNISIAN CHICK PEA SOUP

500 g / 1¼ lb chick peas, soaked overnight in
   cold water
1 litre / 1¾ pints water
2 tablespoons olive oil
1 tablespoon caraway seeds
3 garlic cloves, crushed
1 tablespoon Tahini paste
2 tablespoons lemon juice

SERVES 4–6
4 servings
Per serving: **Energy** 490 kcal / 2060 kJ
           Fat 17 g
           Fibre 19 g
6 servings
Per serving: **Energy** 325 kcal / 1370 kJ
           Fat 11 g
           Fibre 13 g

Drain the chick peas and place in a saucepan with the water. Bring to the boil and boil briskly for 10 minutes. Then reduce the heat, add the oil and caraway seeds and cook gently for about 1¼ hours.

Add the garlic and Tahini paste, blending well. Simmer for a further 25–30 minutes. Stir in the lemon juice and serve hot.

ITALIAN MINESTRONE

½ leek, cleaned and shredded
1 onion, finely chopped
1 garlic clove, crushed
1 tablespoon olive oil
1.2 litres / 2 pints white stock
1 carrot, scrubbed and cut into thin strips
1 turnip, peeled and cut into thin strips
1 celery stick, scrubbed and thinly sliced
25 g / 1 oz wholemeal macaroni
¼ white cabbage, washed and finely shredded
3 runner beans, thinly sliced
25 g / 1 oz shelled peas
1 teaspoon tomato purée
4 tomatoes, diced

1–2 rashers lean bacon, rinded, chopped and
   grilled
freshly ground black pepper
Parmesan cheese, grated

SERVES 4–6
4 servings
Per serving: **Energy** 140 kcal / 585 kJ
           Fat 6 g
           Fibre 6 g
6 servings
Per serving: **Energy** 95 kcal / 390 kJ
           Fat 4 g
           Fibre 4 g

Cook the leek, onion and garlic in the oil for 5–10 minutes, until soft but not coloured. Add the stock, bring to the boil, add the carrot, turnip, celery and macaroni and simmer for 20–30 minutes. Add the cabbage, beans and peas and simmer for a further 20 minutes. Stir in the tomato purée and tomatoes, bacon and seasoning to taste. Serve the Parmesan cheese in a separate dish.

MEDITERRANEAN VEGETABLE SOUP WITH PISTOU

2 tablespoons olive oil
1 medium onion, chopped
2 small leeks, cleaned and chopped
1.2 litres/2 pints hot water
2 small carrots, scrubbed and chopped
150 g/5 oz cooked haricot beans
freshly ground black pepper
175 g/6 oz courgettes, cut in 1 cm/½ inch slices
175 g/6 oz string beans, cut in 2.5 cm/1 inch pieces
225 g/8 oz tomatoes, chopped

75 g/3 oz short wholemeal macaroni
PISTOU
3 garlic cloves, finely chopped
40 g/1½ oz finely chopped basil leaves
25 g/1 oz freshly grated Parmesan cheese
2 tablespoons olive oil

SERVES 8
Per serving: **Energy** 160 kcal/675 kJ
          Fat 9 g
          Fibre 6 g

Heat the oil in a heavy pan and cook the onion and leeks until softened and pale golden. Add the hot water, carrots and haricot beans. (Canned haricot beans may be used as an alternative, in which case add them when the other vegetables are cooked.) Bring to the boil, add pepper and simmer for 45 minutes. Add the courgettes, string beans and tomatoes and simmer for a further 20 minutes. Add the macaroni and cook for about 15 minutes longer, until tender.

While the soup is cooking, make the pistou. Pound the garlic to a pulp in a mortar. Add the basil leaves to the garlic. Pound again until the garlic and basil are amalgamated. Add the grated cheese and continue pounding. When all is smooth, beat in the oil drop by drop. When all has blended into a smooth paste, put the pistou in a warm tureen and pour the boiling soup over it. Cover the tureen and stand for 5 minutes. *Illustrated on p. 11.*

BASIC FISH STOCK

1 kg/2 lb raw white fish (e.g. whiting or turbot)
fish bones, heads and trimmings
1 medium onion, sliced
1 celery stick, sliced
12 peppercorns
1 bay leaf
1 tablespoon lemon juice

rind of 1 lemon
4 parsley stalks
2.25 litres/4 pints cold water
3 tablespoons dry white wine (optional)

MAKES about 2.5 litres/4½ pints
Energy/Fat/Fibre content negligible

Put all the ingredients into a large saucepan. Bring to the boil and skim thoroughly. Simmer for 25 minutes. Strain and cool the liquid.

If a stronger stock is needed, reduce the strained liquid by rapid boiling to half the quantity.

Any surplus stock can be frozen.

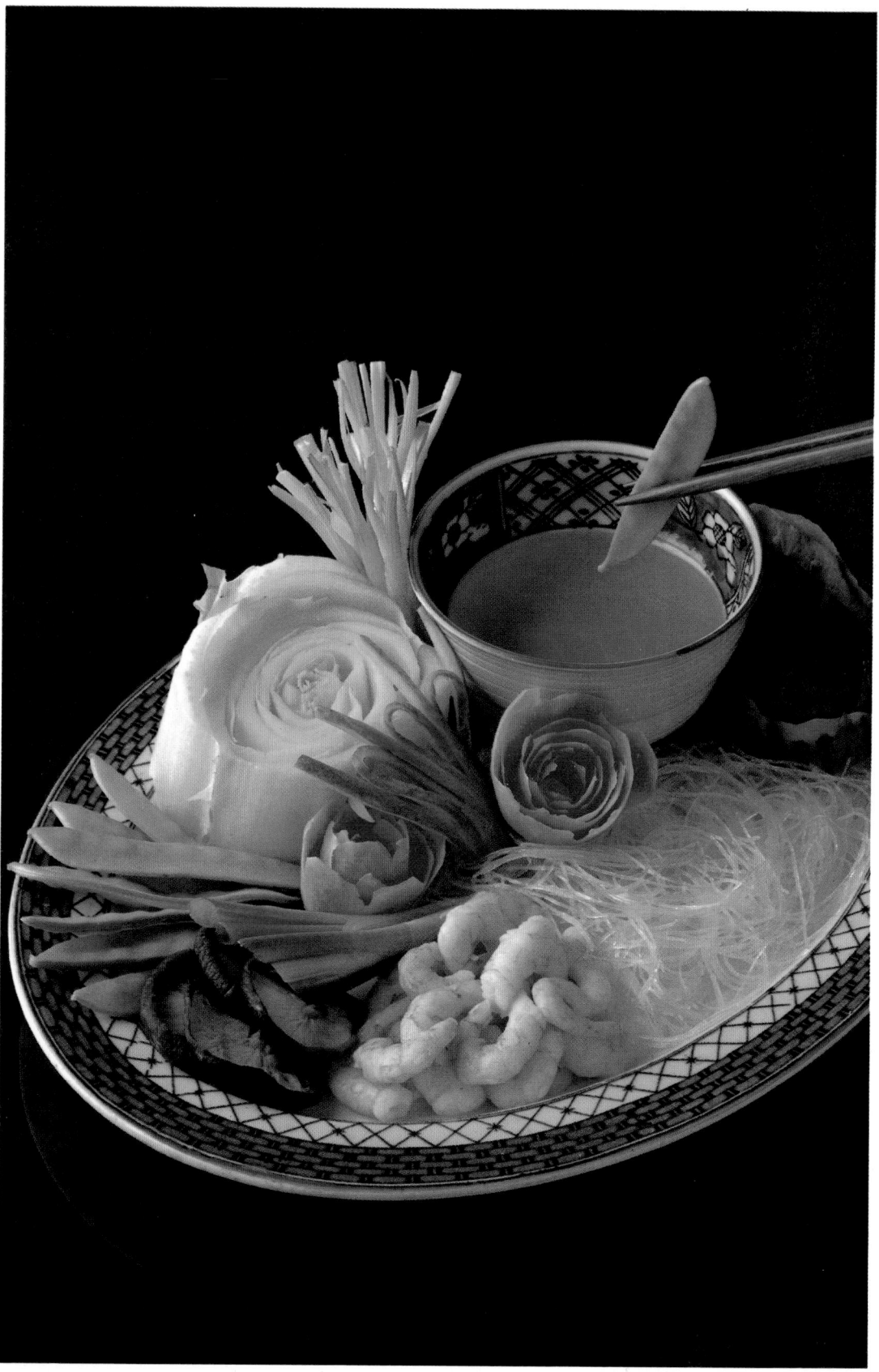

JAPANESE HARUSAME SOUP

100 g/4 oz dehydrated mung bean threads (saifun) or soy bean noodles, soaked in boiling water for 30 minutes
2–3 dried mushrooms, soaked in boiling water for 20 minutes
1 litre/1¾ pints chicken stock
1 tablespoon rice wine
100 g/4 oz peeled fresh or frozen prawns
6–8 mangetout
2 carrots, scrubbed and sliced or chopped
few cucumber strips

100 g/4 oz celery or Chinese cabbage (napa)
few spinach leaves
TO GARNISH
1 teaspoon grated fresh root ginger
1 spring onion, finely shredded
2 teaspoons puréed white radish (daikon)

SERVES 4
Per serving: **Energy** 140 kcal/595 kJ
Fat 5 g
Fibre 2 g

Drain the mung bean threads or soy bean noodles and cut into 5 cm/2 inch lengths. Drain the mushrooms, reserving the soaking liquid; cut off the stems.

Put the stock in a saucepan. Pour in the mushroom soaking liquid carefully, discarding any sandy sediment at the bottom. Bring to the boil and simmer for 2 min-utes. Stir in the rice wine.

Divide the liquid between 4 warmed soup bowls. Arrange the remaining ingred ients on a serving dish, cutting the veget ables to make attractive shapes, if wished. Place the garnish ingredients on separate dishes. Each person adds ingredients and garnishes to his bowl, according to taste.

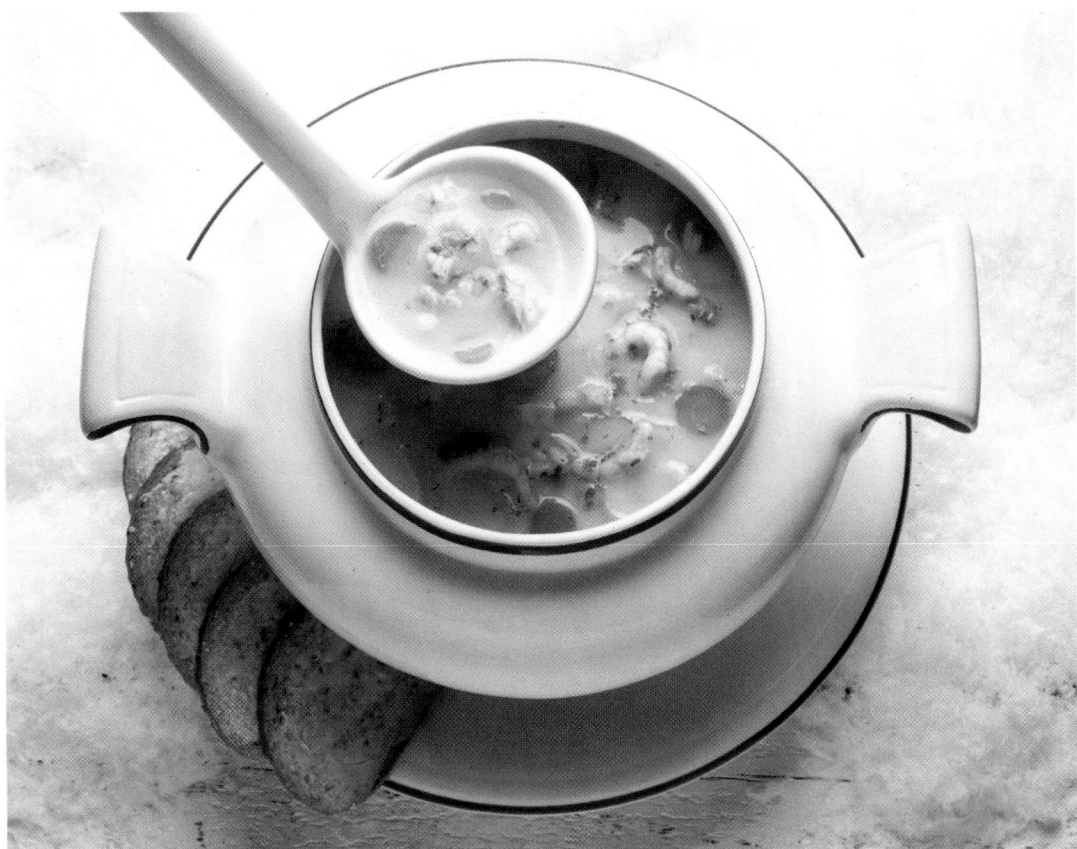

OPPOSITE: JAPANESE HARUSAME SOUP.   ABOVE: SCANDINAVIAN SALMON SOUP (P.44)

SCANDINAVIAN SALMON SOUP

75 g/3 oz long-grain brown rice
the head of a large salmon, washed
1.2 litres/2 pints Basic fish stock (page 41)
1 onion, sliced
2 carrots, scrubbed and thinly sliced
1 celery stick, thinly sliced
½ teaspoon dill seeds
freshly ground black pepper

TO GARNISH
few peeled shrimps
chopped fresh dill or parsley

SERVES 4

Per serving:	**Energy**	125 kcal/530 kJ
	Fat	4 g
	Fibre	2 g

A friendly fishmonger will let you have a large salmon head relatively cheaply. Rye bread goes well with this impressive soup.

Put the rice in a strainer, rinse well under cold running water then leave to drain. Place the salmon head in a large pan and pour in the stock. Bring to the boil, reduce the heat, then simmer gently for 20 minutes. Remove the head on to a dish. Strain the liquid into a clean pan, then add the rice, onion, carrots, celery, dill seeds and pepper to taste. Bring to the boil, reduce the heat, then simmer for about 20 minutes, or until the rice and vegetables are tender.

Meanwhile, pick the flesh from the fish head and add to the soup. Reheat gently, then taste and adjust the seasoning. Pour into a heated tureen or individual soup dishes and garnish with shrimps and dill. *Illustrated on p. 43.*

BORTSCH

1.75 litres/3 pints chicken or beef stock
100 g/4 oz white cabbage, finely shredded and
  chopped
1 carrot, scrubbed and finely chopped
1 onion, finely chopped
1 celery stick, scrubbed and finely chopped
450 g/1 lb raw beetroot, peeled
1 tablespoon chopped fresh parsley
2 cloves
1 bay leaf
2 tomatoes, chopped
2 teaspoons caster sugar
2 tablespoons lemon juice

freshly ground black pepper
150 ml/5 oz plain unsweetened yogurt

SERVES 8–10

8 servings

Per serving:	**Energy**	40 kcal/165 kJ
	Fat	1 g
	Fibre	3 g

10 servings

Per serving:	**Energy**	30 kcal/130 kJ
	Fat	1 g
	Fibre	2 g

This traditional Russian soup should be thick with vegetables cut small so that they fit easily on to a soup spoon. If you have a blender, you can prepare the beetroot cleanly by putting it into the goblet, a little at a time, with some of the stock and quickly chopping it to size. Alternatively, the beetroot can be coarsely grated.

Put the stock into a large pan with the cabbage, carrot, onion and celery. Prepare the beetroot and add three-quarters to the stock with the parsley, cloves and bay leaf. Bring to the boil, then cover and simmer for 30 minutes.

Add the tomatoes, sugar, lemon juice and pepper and simmer for a further 20 minutes. To ensure the soup is a good red colour, stir in the remaining beetroot, then simmer for a further 10 minutes. Serve the bortsch hot with a spoonful of yogurt dropped into each bowl.

FRENCH FABONADE

2 teaspoons olive oil
1 small onion, finely chopped
2 rashers lean bacon, rinded and diced
4 garlic cloves, crushed
1 kg/2 lb broad beans, shelled
150 ml/¼ pint water
few sprigs savory
freshly ground black pepper
2 egg yolks
1 teaspoon wine vinegar or lemon juice

TO GARNISH
chopped parsley

SERVES 4
Per serving: **Energy** 190 kcal/795 kJ
               Fat 7 g
               Fibre 11 g

Heat the oil in a heavy pan, add the onion and bacon and cook gently for a few minutes. Add the garlic and beans, then the water, savory, and pepper to taste. Mix well.

Bring to the boil, then lower the heat, cover and simmer for 20–30 minutes until the beans are tender.

Discard the savory. Mix the egg yolks and vinegar or lemon juice together, then stir slowly into the beans. Heat through, but do not allow to boil. Taste and adjust seasoning, then transfer to a warmed serving dish and garnish with parsley. Serve immediately.

INDIAN NIRAMISH VEGETABLES

350 g/12 oz cauliflower florets
175 g/6 oz carrots, scrubbed
225 g/8 oz potatoes, unpeeled
5–6 tablespoons corn oil
½ teaspoon panch-phoran (mixture of cumin, fennel, fenugreek, mustard and onion seeds)
1 large onion, finely chopped
½ teaspoon ground turmeric
175 g/6 oz frozen green beans, thawed and chopped
175 g/6 oz frozen peas
2 medium tomatoes, sliced
1 teaspoon lemon juice

SERVES 6–8
6 servings
Per serving: **Energy** 340 kcal/1425 kJ
               Fat 30 g
               Fibre 6 g
8 servings
Per serving: **Energy** 255 kcal/1070 kJ
               Fat 23 g
               Fibre 5 g

If you eat Indian food frequently, it is worth buying quantities of the different spices used in panch-phoran and making up a blend to store in a glass-stoppered jar.

Steam the cauliflower, carrots and potatoes until they are almost cooked but still firm in the centre. Peel the potatoes and cut into rough cubes. Cut the carrots into slices about 5 mm/¼ inch thick.

Heat the oil in a heavy frying pan. Take the pan off the heat and add the panch-phoran. Cover with a lid because the seeds will start to burst. Leave for ½ minute, then remove the lid and put the pan back over a low heat. Add the onion and fry until lightly browned. Add the turmeric. Leave for 1 minute, then add the par-cooked vegetables and green beans and fry for 3–4 minutes, stirring frequently to break them up. Add the peas, tomatoes and lemon juice. Leave over a very low heat for a further 2–3 minutes.

FRENCH FÈVES EN RAGOÛT

1 tablespoon olive oil
1 kg/2 lb broad beans, shelled
2 garlic cloves, crushed
75 g/3 oz lean bacon, rinded, lightly grilled and
    diced
150 ml/¼ pint water
3 carrots, scrubbed and cut into thin rounds
6 small pickling onions, peeled
1 bouquet garni

1 sprig savory
pinch of caster sugar
freshly ground black pepper

SERVES 6
Per serving: **Energy** 105 kcal/445 kJ
                 Fat 4 g
                 Fibre 8 g

Heat the oil in a heavy pan, add the beans and garlic. Cook gently for a few minutes, stirring constantly, then add the remaining ingredients with pepper to taste. Mix well.

Bring to the boil, lower the heat, cover and simmer for 20–30 minutes until the beans are tender. Discard the bouquet garni and savory, then taste and adjust seasoning. Transfer to a warmed serving dish and serve immediately.

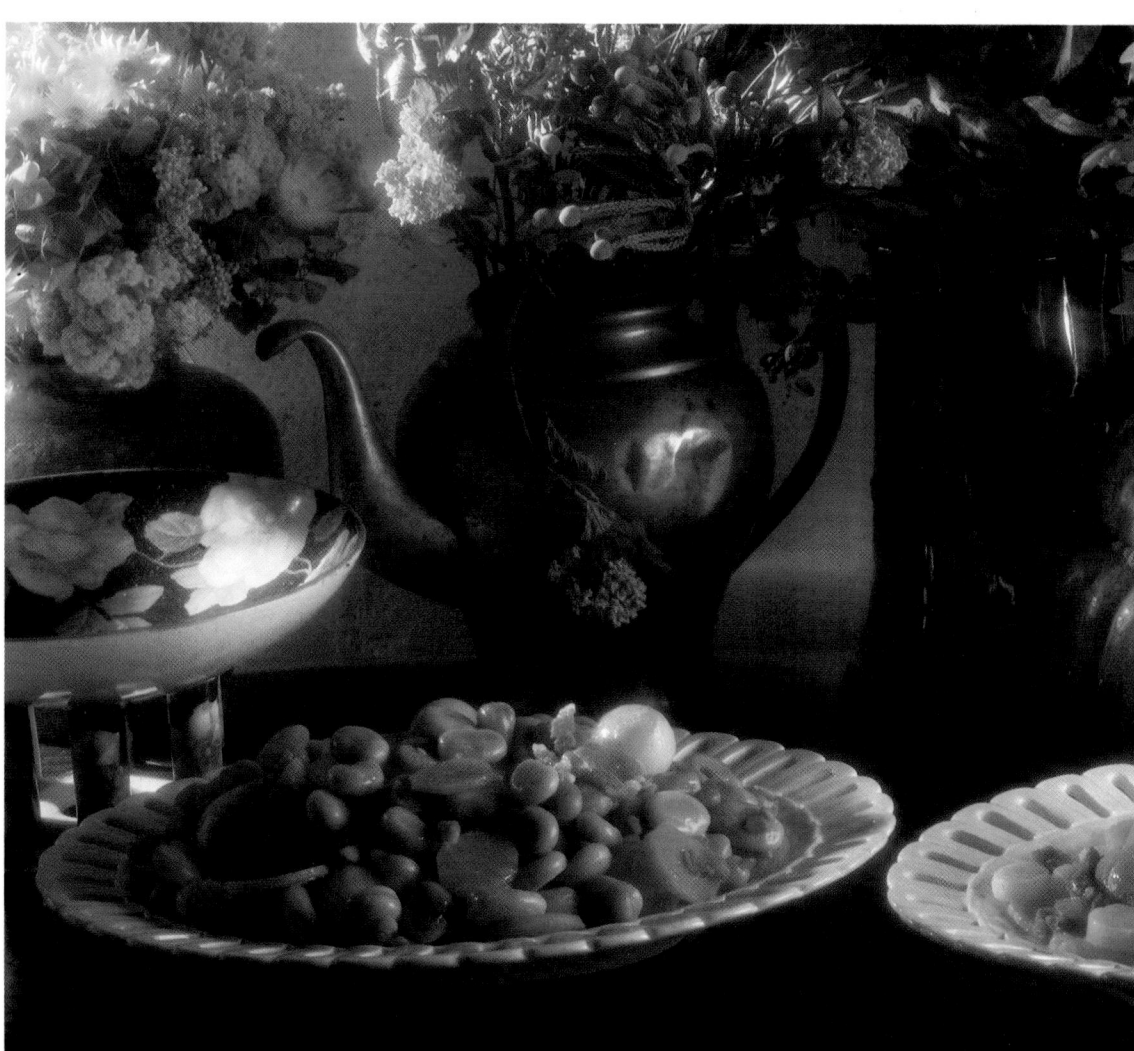

FRENCH PORROSALDA

750 g / 1½ lb potatoes, peeled and sliced into rounds
1 kg / 2 lb leeks (white part only), sliced into rings
3 tablespoons plain wholemeal flour
450 ml / ¾ pint vegetable stock or water
50 g / 2 oz lean bacon, lightly grilled and diced
2 garlic cloves, crushed

1 bouquet garni
freshly ground black pepper

SERVES 6
Per serving: **Energy** 195 kcal/825 kJ
           Fat   2 g
           Fibre 9 g

Put the potatoes and leeks in a large heavy pan. Combine the flour and stock or water and pour over the vegetables. Add the bacon, garlic, bouquet garni and pepper to taste. Cover and simmer gently for about 30 minutes or until the potatoes are tender.

Discard the bouquet garni, then taste and adjust seasoning.

Transfer the porrosalda to a warmed serving dish and serve immediately.

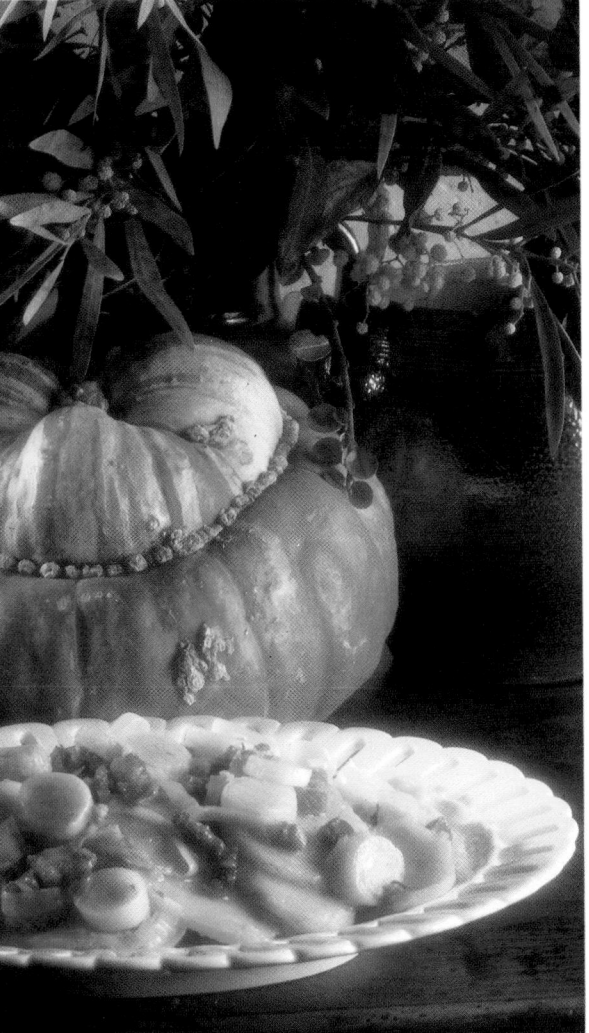

VIENNESE LENTIL SALAD

350 g / 12 oz green lentils, soaked in cold water for 1 hour
freshly ground black pepper
1 garlic clove, finely chopped
2 spring onions, chopped
4 tablespoons Apple juice dressing (page 58)
4 rashers lean bacon, rinded, crisply grilled and diced

SERVES 4
Per serving: **Energy** 380 kcal/1590 kJ
           Fat   10 g
           Fibre 11 g

Place the lentils in a pan, cover with cold water, bring to the boil and cook for about 50 minutes or until tender. Drain, rinse under cold water and place in a serving bowl. Season to taste with pepper. Stir in the garlic and onions.

Pour the dressing over the lentil mixture and toss thoroughly. Sprinkle the diced bacon over, or stir into the salad, as liked. Serve immediately. *Illustrated on p. 60.*

FAR LEFT: FÈVES EN RAGOÛT; LEFT: FRENCH PORROSALDA

GREEK BEAN SALAD

275 g / 10 oz dried black-eye or white haricot
    beans, soaked overnight in cold water
1 litre / 1¾ pints water
cayenne pepper
4 tomatoes, diced
2 large onions, chopped
100 g / 4 oz Feta cheese, cubed
2 garlic cloves, crushed

1 tablespoon wine vinegar
3 tablespoons olive oil
½ teaspoon chopped oregano leaves

SERVES 4

Per serving:	Energy	335 kcal / 1340 kJ
	Fat	17 g
	Fibre	16 g

If fresh oregano is unobtainable, use chopped parsley instead.

Drain the beans and place in a pan with water. Bring to the boil and boil rapidly for 10 minutes. Then lower the heat and cook gently for about 1 hour. Season to taste with cayenne pepper and cook for a further 10–20 minutes, until just tender. Drain in a sieve and leave to cool.

Place the beans in a large serving bowl and mix with the tomatoes, onions and cheese.

To make the dressing, beat the garlic with the vinegar, olive oil and oregano. Pour over the salad and toss to mix.

Leave to stand for 10–15 minutes to allow the flavours to develop. Toss again before serving. *Illustrated on p. 60.*

SARDINIAN SEAFOOD SALAD

225 g / 8 oz wholemeal macaroni
100 g / 4 oz cooked and shelled mussels
100 g / 4 oz peeled fresh or frozen prawns
1 × 50 g (2 oz) can anchovies, drained and
    wiped
50 g / 2 oz mushrooms, thinly sliced
4 tomatoes, cut into wedges
3 tablespoons Apple juice dressing (page 58)
2 tablespoons tomato juice
½ teaspoon dried oregano

TO GARNISH
2 tablespoons chopped fresh parsley
1 tablespoon grated Parmesan cheese
4 lemon twists

SERVES 4

Per serving:	Energy	335 kcal / 1395 kJ
	Fat	10 g
	Fibre	7 g

Cook the macaroni in a large pan of boiling water for 10 minutes until tender but *al dente*. Drain thoroughly.

While still warm, mix the pasta with the mussels, prawns and anchovies. Add the mushrooms and tomatoes. Combine the dressing with the tomato juice and oregano. Pour over the pasta mixture. Mix thoroughly and turn into a serving dish. Chill in the refrigerator for 2 hours.

Sprinkle over the chopped parsley and Parmesan cheese and garnish with lemon twists. Serve immediately.

OPPOSITE: SARDINIAN SEAFOOD SALAD

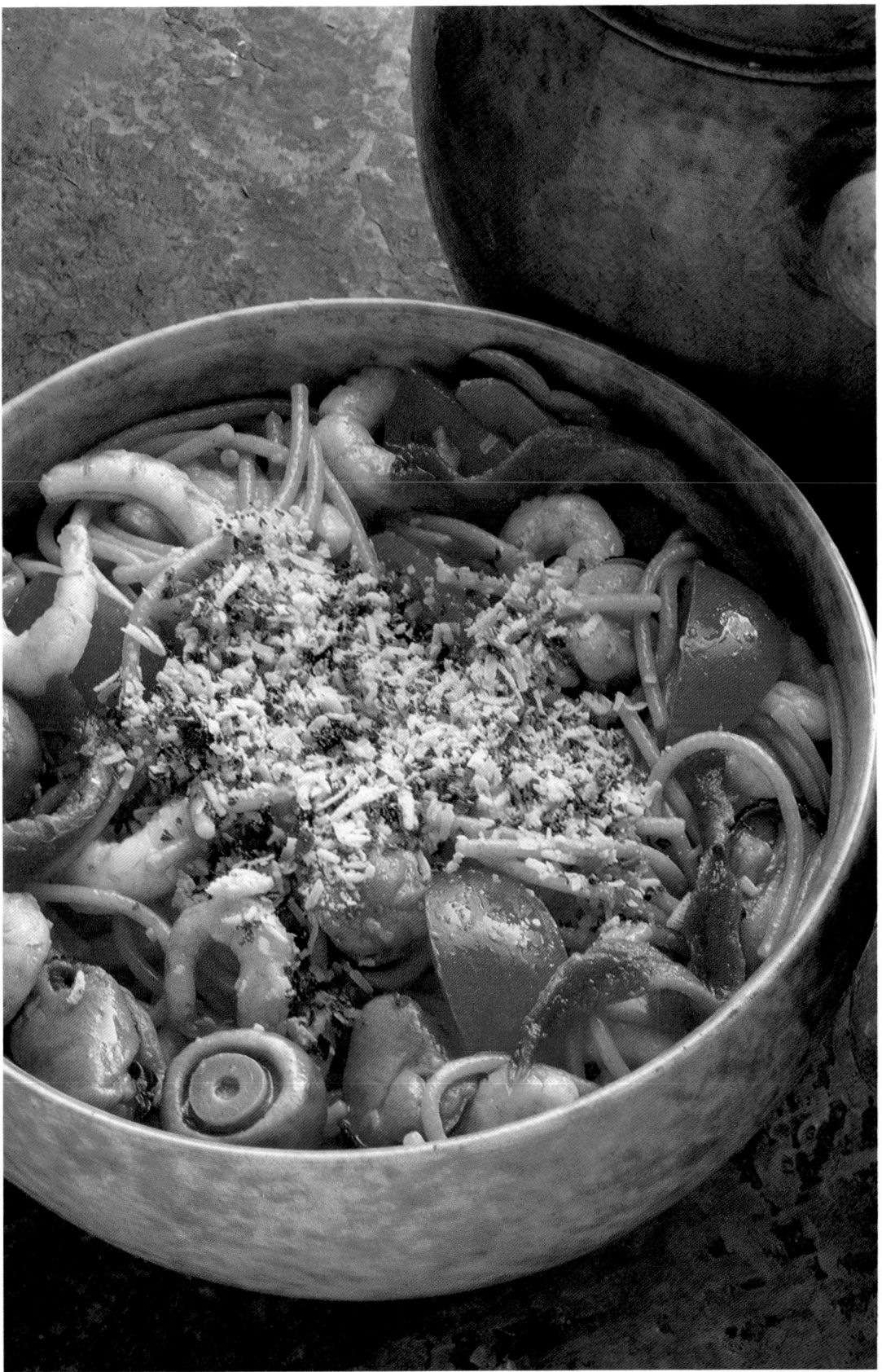

AMERICAN SUCCOTASH SALAD

225 g/8 oz broad beans, fresh or frozen
225 g/8 oz sweetcorn kernels, fresh or frozen
150 ml/¼ pint Sesame dressing (page 58)
4 large crisp lettuce leaves
TO GARNISH
chopped parsley

SERVES 4
Per serving: **Energy** 200 kcal/835 kJ
Fat 12 g
Fibre 7 g

Put the broad beans and sweetcorn into a saucepan half-filled with boiling water. Simmer for about 10 minutes or until the beans are tender. Drain thoroughly and leave to cool.

Mix the vegetables with the dressing and arrange the mixture on lettuce leaves on individual plates. Garnish with parsley.

JAPANESE SASHIMI

750 g/1½ lb fresh sea bass, tuna or other
saltwater fish, filleted
175 g/6 oz white radish (daikon), shredded
4–5 spring onions, shredded
175 g/6 oz mangetout
few cooked giant prawns in shell
1 tablespoon ground green horseradish (wasabi)
lemon wedges

1 tablespoon grated fresh root ginger
light soy sauce to taste

SERVES 4
Per serving: **Energy** 250 kcal/1060 kJ
Fat 5 g
Fibre 1 g

Remove any skin, bones and dark sections from the fish. Cut it diagonally into slices 2.5 cm/1 inch long and 5 mm/¼ inch thick.

Arrange the slices of fish on a platter with the vegetables and prawns. Mix the horseradish to a thick paste with a little water and place on the platter with lemon wedges and the ginger. Pour soy sauce into small individual bowls.

Each person adds horseradish and ginger to his bowl of soy sauce, then uses this as a dip for the fish and vegetables.

JAPANESE PIQUANT PORK AND PRAWNS WITH VERMICELLI

275 g/10 oz thin wholemeal vermicelli
1 tablespoon olive oil
1 garlic clove, crushed
1 medium onion, thinly sliced
175 g/6 oz lean pork, cut into strips 5 cm/2
inches long and 1 cm/½ inch wide
75 g/3 oz fresh prawns, peeled and chopped
freshly ground black pepper
1 tablespoon light soy sauce
2 tablespoons tomato purée
1 teaspoon grated lemon rind
2 tablespoons lemon juice

3 tablespoons unsalted peanuts
4 tablespoons finely chopped spring onions
2 medium oranges, peeled and sliced
TO GARNISH
1 slice orange
watercress

SERVES 6
Per serving: **Energy** 320 kcal/1350 kJ
Fat 11 g
Fibre 7 g

Cook the vermicelli in boiling water until just tender. Drain well. Meanwhile heat the oil in a large frying pan. Add the garlic and fry until golden brown. Discard the garlic. Add the onion and pork and fry until the onion is softened and the pork begins to change colour. Stir in the prawns and pepper to taste and continue cooking,

stirring constantly, for 3 minutes.

Add the soy sauce, tomato purée, lemon rind and juice, peanuts, spring onions and orange slices. Add the vermicelli to the pan. Continue cooking, tossing and stirring lightly, until piping hot. Transfer to a serving dish and garnish with orange and watercress.

CHINESE CHICKEN AND BEAN-SPROUTS

225 g/8 oz chicken breast meat, boned and
  skinned
1 egg white
1 tablespoon cornflour
225 g/8 oz fresh bean-sprouts
1 small red pepper, cored, seeded and cut into
  thin shreds

3 tablespoons olive oil
2 tablespoons chicken stock

SERVES 4
Per serving: Energy 205 kcal/870 kJ
                Fat   14 g
                Fibre 2 g

Slice the chicken meat into slivers not much bigger than a matchstick. Mix the slivers with the egg white and then the cornflour, in that order.

Wash the bean-sprouts in a basin of cold water, discarding the husks and any little bits that float to the surface (it is not necessary to top and tail each sprout).

Heat the oil in a wok or frying pan and

stir-fry the chicken pieces until lightly coloured, then remove them with a perforated spoon.

Increase the heat and when the oil is hot, add the bean-sprouts and red pepper followed by the chicken. Stir a few times, then add the stock. Cook for about 1 minute more.

This dish may be served hot or cold.

MEDITERRANEAN GRATIN

225 g/8 oz lean ground beef
1 medium onion, chopped
1 garlic clove, crushed
225 g/8 oz courgettes, sliced
1 aubergine, diced
1 × 400 g (14 oz) can tomatoes
1/2 teaspoon dried thyme
1/2 teaspoon dried rosemary
freshly ground black pepper

200 g/7 oz long-grain brown rice
600 ml/1 pint beef stock
2 tablespoons grated Parmesan cheese
2 tablespoons wholemeal breadcrumbs

SERVES 4
Per serving: Energy 330 kcal/1385 kJ
                Fat   7 g
                Fibre 6 g

Fry the beef gently in a large frying pan without additional fat until browned. Add the onion, garlic, courgettes and aubergine. Add the tomatoes together with the herbs and pepper to taste. Mix well, cover and simmer for 35 minutes.

Put the rice and stock into a saucepan. Bring to the boil and stir once. Lower heat

to simmer, cover and cook for 15 minutes, or until rice is tender and liquid absorbed. Mix the rice with the vegetable and meat mixture and place in a shallow ovenproof dish, sprinkle with the cheese and breadcrumbs and place under a preheated grill for 10 minutes.

Serve the gratin hot.

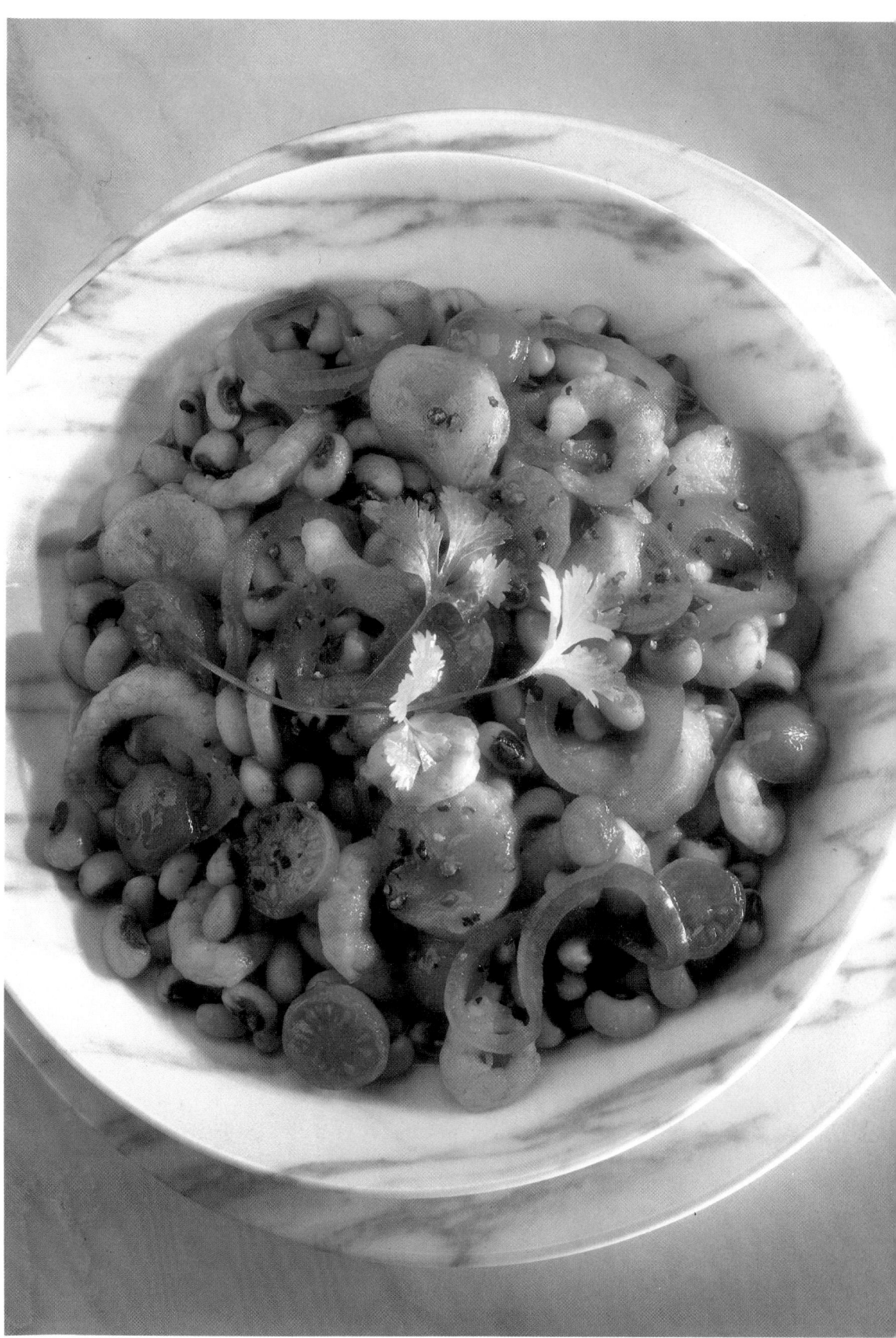

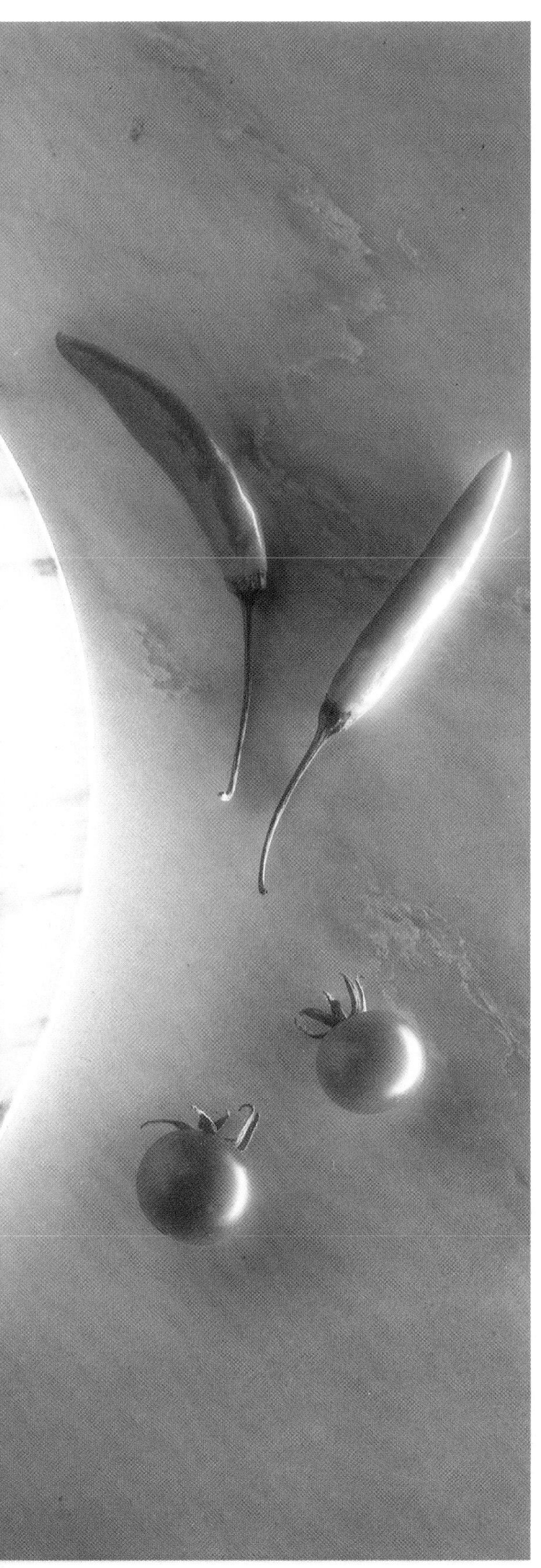

WEST AFRICAN PRAWNS AND BLACK-EYE BEANS

200 g / 7 oz black-eye beans, soaked overnight in
cold water
about 600 ml / 1 pint water
1½ tablespoons corn oil
1 medium onion, sliced into rings
½ teaspoon chilli powder
2 teaspoons tomato purée
400 g / 14 oz cherry tomatoes, halved
150 g / 5 oz fresh or frozen prawns
2 large bananas, sliced
TO GARNISH
fresh coriander leaves

SERVES 4
Per serving: **Energy** 325 kcal / 1360 kJ
                Fat 8 g
                Fibre 15 g

Drain the beans and put into a saucepan with the water. Bring to the boil and boil rapidly for 10 minutes. Then simmer for about 25 minutes until tender, adding a little more water if necessary.

Heat the oil and cook the onion until golden. Add the chili powder and tomato purée and cook for a few minutes. Add this mixture to the beans and simmer for 20 minutes. Add the tomatoes and prawns and simmer very gently for a further 10 minutes, adding the bananas in the last 5 minutes.

Serve garnished with fresh coriander leaves.

WEST INDIAN TUNA FISH RISOTTO

225 g/8 oz long-grain brown rice
2 tablespoons olive oil
2 medium onions, chopped
1 green pepper, cored, seeded and chopped
2 teaspoons curry powder
200 g/7 oz ground unsalted peanuts
450 ml/¾ pint apple juice
2 tablespoons lemon juice
1 dessert apple, peeled, cored and diced

1 tablespoon caster sugar
freshly ground black pepper
2 × 200 g (7 oz) cans tuna fish, drained, wiped and flaked

SERVES 6

Per serving:	Energy	565 kcal/2285 kJ
	Fat	33 g
	Fibre	5 g

Cook the rice in boiling water for 10 minutes. Drain well.

Heat the oil in a large saucepan. Add the onions and green pepper and cook until softened. Stir in the curry powder and cook for 2 minutes, then add the peanuts, apple and lemon juices, apple, sugar and pepper. Bring to the boil, stirring well.

Stir in the rice and tuna and simmer for 10 minutes or until the rice is tender.

MEXICAN TUNA BEAN APPETIZER

3 eating apples, cored and chopped
1 tablespoon lemon juice
1 × 90 g (3½ oz) can tuna fish, drained, wiped and flaked
1 small onion, finely chopped
3 celery sticks, thinly sliced
2 tablespoons chopped green olives

1 × 425 g (15 oz) can red kidney beans, drained
2 tablespoons Apple juice dressing (page 58)

SERVES 4

Per serving:	Energy	190 kcal/800 kJ
	Fat	10 g
	Fibre	7 g

Coat the apples with the lemon juice to prevent discoloration. Place in a bowl with the tuna, onion, celery, olives and beans.

Add the dressing and toss well.

Chill the dish in the refrigerator for 30 minutes before serving.

TABBOULEH

225 g/8 oz cracked wheat, soaked for 30-45 minutes in cold water
3 tablespoons finely chopped onion
freshly ground black pepper
2 tablespoons sesame oil
5 tablespoons lemon or lime juice
3 tablespoons finely chopped fresh mint
6 tablespoons finely chopped fresh parsley
½ cucumber, finely chopped
½ cos lettuce
TO GARNISH
black olives, stoned

SERVES 4–6
4 servings

Per serving:	Energy	260 kcal/1095 kJ
	Fat	9 g
	Fibre	2 g

6 servings

Per serving:	Energy	175 kcal/730 kJ
	Fat	6 g
	Fibre	1 g

Drain the cracked wheat and squeeze out as much moisture as possible in a clean teatowel.

Mix the cracked wheat and onion by hand, squeezing the mixture to extract the onion juice. Season with pepper. Add the sesame oil, lemon or lime juice and herbs.

Set aside for 15 minutes to allow flavours to develop. Stir well and taste – it may need more lemon or lime juice or black pepper.

Add the cucumber just before serving and arrange individual portions on lettuce leaves. Garnish each portion of tabbouleh with black olives.

NORTH AFRICAN CHAKCHOUKA

2 tablespoons olive oil
2 medium onions, sliced
1/2 teaspoon chilli powder
2 red peppers, cored, seeded and thinly sliced
2 green peppers, cored, seeded and thinly sliced
6 tomatoes, chopped
freshly ground black pepper
8 eggs

SERVES 4
Per serving: **Energy** 365 kcal/1525 kJ
                Fat 19 g
                Fibre 2 g

Heat the oil in frying pan. Add the onions and fry until softened. Stir in the chilli powder and fry for 1 minute, then add the red and green peppers, tomatoes and pepper to taste. Cover and cook for 10 minutes.

Divide the vegetable mixture between 4 shallow baking dishes and make two hollows in each. Break the eggs into the hollows and season with pepper.

Cook in a preheated moderately hot oven (200°C, 400°F, Gas Mark 6) for 8–10 minutes or until the eggs are set. Serve hot with crusty wholemeal rolls.

ITALIAN SPINACH GNOCCHI

450 g/1 lb fresh spinach, or 1 × 400 g (14 oz)
   packet frozen spinach
100 g/4 oz cottage cheese
freshly ground black pepper
1 teaspoon grated nutmeg
25 g/1 oz grated Parmesan cheese
1 egg
40 g/1 1/2 oz plain wholemeal flour

SERVES 4
Per serving: **Energy** 135 kcal/560 kJ
                Fat 5 g
                Fibre 8 g

Cook the spinach in a very little boiling water in a covered pan. Drain, squeeze and chop finely. Sieve the cottage cheese. Return the spinach to the pan with the pepper, nutmeg and cottage cheese. Stir over a low heat for 5 minutes. Remove from the heat and beat in half the Parmesan cheese, the egg and flour. Turn on to a plate and flatten. Leave to cool for several hours.

Using a little flour, shape the mixture into small croquettes. Have ready a large pan of boiling water, drop the spinach gnocchi into it and cook for approximately 5 minutes. When they are cooked they will rise to the top. Drain the gnocchi in a colander. Place in an ovenproof dish which has been lightly oiled and sprinkled with Parmesan cheese. Dredge the gnocchi with the remaining Parmesan cheese and warm in a preheated moderate oven (180°C, 350°F, Gas Mark 4) for 5 minutes.

RATATOUILLE NICOISE

85 ml / 3 fl oz olive oil
450 g / 1 lb aubergines, thinly sliced or diced
450 g / 1 lb courgettes, sliced
450 g / 1 lb onions, thinly sliced
450 g / 1 lb green peppers, cored, seeded and cut
into thin strips
5 garlic cloves, crushed

750 g / 1½ lb tomatoes, halved
freshly ground black pepper
2 sprigs thyme
basil leaves
TO GARNISH
chopped parsley

SERVES 6–8
6 servings

Per serving:	**Energy**	195 kcal/820 kJ
	Fat	15 g
	Fibre	7 g

8 servings

Per serving:	**Energy**	145 kcal/615 kJ
	Fat	11 g
	Fibre	5 g

Heat half the oil in a large heavy pan, add the aubergines and cook over a moderate heat until lightly coloured, stirring frequently. Add the courgettes and continue cooking for 5–6 minutes until they are lightly coloured. Remove both aubergines and courgettes with a slotted spoon and set aside.

Add the remaining oil to the pan, then add the onions and cook gently until soft. Add the peppers and garlic, increase the heat and cook for a few minutes. Add the tomatoes and cook gently for 10 minutes, stirring frequently.

Return the aubergines and courgettes to the pan and stir well to mix with the other vegetables. Add pepper to taste, then crumble in the thyme. Cook gently, uncovered, for 40 minutes or until the vegetables are soft, stirring occasionally.

Just before serving, crumble the basil leaves into the ratatouille, then taste and adjust seasoning. Transfer to a warmed serving dish and sprinkle with parsley. Serve hot or cold.

RUSSIAN KISSEL

2½ tablespoons cornflour
2 tablespoons dry white wine
1 tablespoon lemon juice
450 ml / ¾ pint fruit purée (redcurrants,
cherries, strawberries or other fruit may be
used)
2–3 teaspoons caster sugar

SERVES 4

Per serving:	**Energy**	60 kcal/240 kJ
	Fat	negligible
	Fibre	2 g

Mix together the cornflour, wine and lemon juice. Bring the fruit purée with the sugar to the boil and stir in the wine mixture. Simmer, stirring constantly, until thickened. Cool, then chill in the refrigerator before serving.

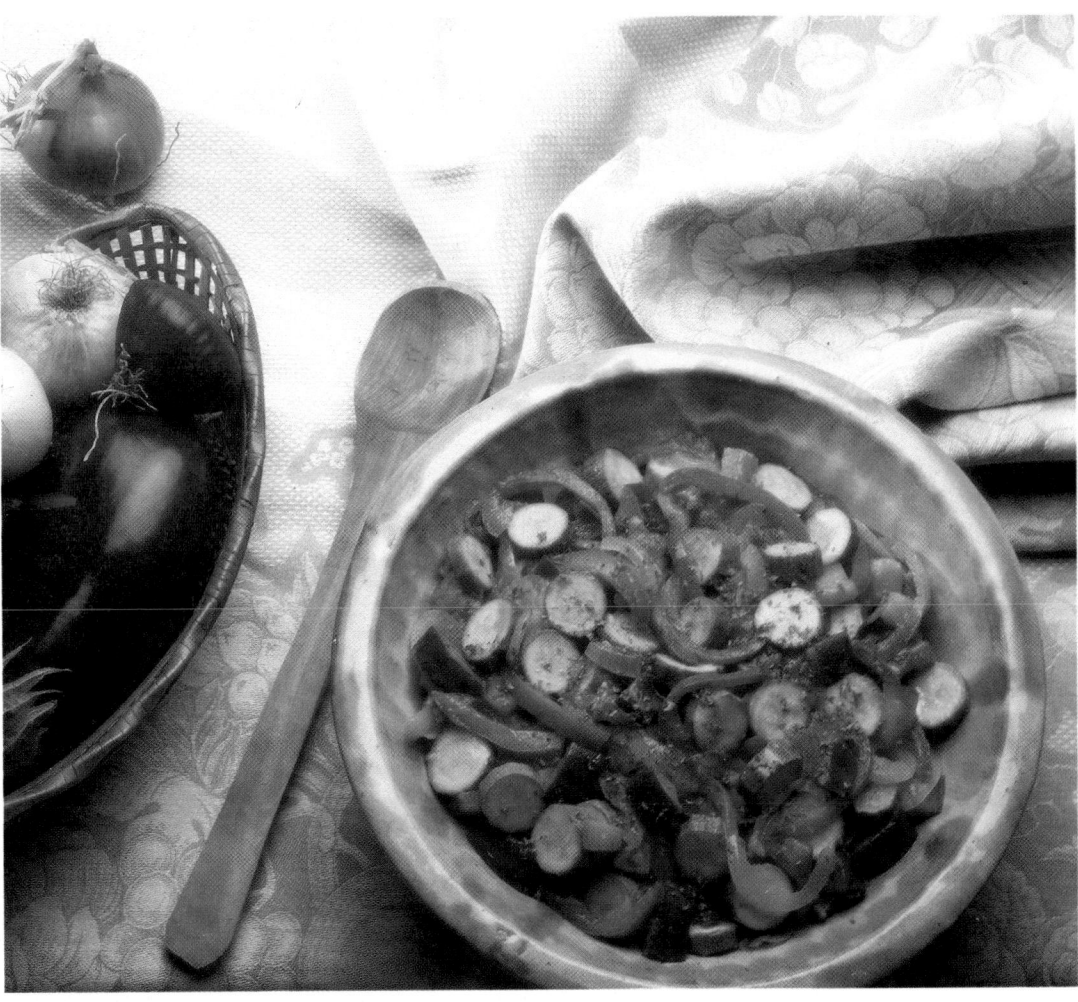

RATATOUILLE NIÇOISE

AMERICAN CRANBERRY RELISH

1 large sweet orange, scrubbed
½ small lemon, scrubbed
300 g / 11 oz fresh cranberries, washed
100 g / 4 oz muscovado sugar

MAKES about 450 g / 1 lb
Total recipe: **Energy** 815 kcal / 3425 kJ
               Fat negligible
               Fibre 16 g

Slice the orange and lemon roughly and remove the pips. If possible, use a food processor to dice the cranberries, orange and lemon; otherwise grind in a food mill. Mix with the sugar. Leave in a refrigerator overnight to allow the flavour to develop.

The relish can be stored in a refrigerator for 3–4 days.

Salads

APPLE JUICE DRESSING

150 ml / ¼ pint olive oil
150 ml / ¼ pint unsweetened apple juice
1 tablespoon lemon juice
1 garlic clove, crushed (optional)
freshly ground black pepper

MAKES about 300 ml / ½ pint
Total volume:

Energy	1415 kcal / 5945 kJ
Fat	150 g
Fibre	negligible

Combine all the ingredients and pour into a screw-topped jar. Shake well before using.

SESAME DRESSING

175 g / 6 oz sesame seeds
400 ml / 14 fl oz water
2–3 garlic cloves, crushed
4 tablespoons lemon juice

MAKES about 300 ml / ½ pint
Total volume:

Energy	1010 kcal / 4280 kJ
Fat	90 g
Fibre	9 g

Put the sesame seeds and water in a blender and blend at maximum speed for 1 minute. Add the remaining ingredients and blend for a further minute.

YOGURT DRESSING

175 ml / 6 fl oz plain unsweetened yogurt
1 tablespoon olive oil
1 teaspoon lemon juice
freshly ground black pepper

MAKES about 200 ml / ⅓ pint
Total volume:

Energy	230 kcal / 950 kJ
Fat	17 g
Fibre	negligible

Combine all the ingredients.

VARIATION
Add 1 teaspoon chopped fresh herbs (mint, chives, basil or thyme).

APRICOT SALAD

175 g/6 oz chicory
350 g/12 oz ripe apricots, stoned
3 celery sticks, diced
75 g/3 oz green olives, chopped
75 g/3 oz flaked almonds
4 tablespoons Yogurt dressing (opposite)

SERVES 4
Per serving: **Energy** 165 kcal/685 kJ
Fat 12 g
Fibre 10 g

Reserve some of the outer leaves of the chicory and slice the remainder thinly. Arrange the reserved whole chicory leaves in a shallow dish.

Mix all the ingredients together and spoon into the dish, on top of the chicory leaves.

PLUM SALAD

750 g/1½ lb ripe dessert plums, stoned
2 teaspoons lemon juice
1 egg
3 tablespoons tarragon wine vinegar
TO GARNISH
1 teaspoon chopped fresh tarragon (optional)

SERVES 4
Per serving: **Energy** 90 kcal/380 kJ
Fat 1 g
Fibre 4 g

Put the plums into a dish and sprinkle with lemon juice. Beat the egg lightly and put into the top of a double saucepan with the vinegar. Cook over a moderate heat, stir-ring constantly, until the mixture thickens. Toss the plums in the warm dressing.

Garnish the dish with tarragon, if liked, before serving.

AVOCADO, GRAPEFRUIT AND SESAME SALAD

2 large avocados
2 tablespoons lemon juice
2 grapefruit, peel and pith removed and
    segmented
1 tablespoon chopped fresh mint
1 small lettuce
2 tablespoons sesame seeds

TO GARNISH
mint sprigs

SERVES 4
Per serving: **Energy** 170 kcal/710 kJ
Fat 15 g
Fibre 2 g

Peel the avocados, cut in half lengthways, then remove the stones. Slice the pulp, place in a bowl, then sprinkle with the lemon juice. Fold in the grapefruit and the chopped mint.

Arrange the lettuce leaves in individual serving bowls. Divide the salad between them, then sprinkle with the sesame seeds. Garnish with sprigs of mint and serve immediately.

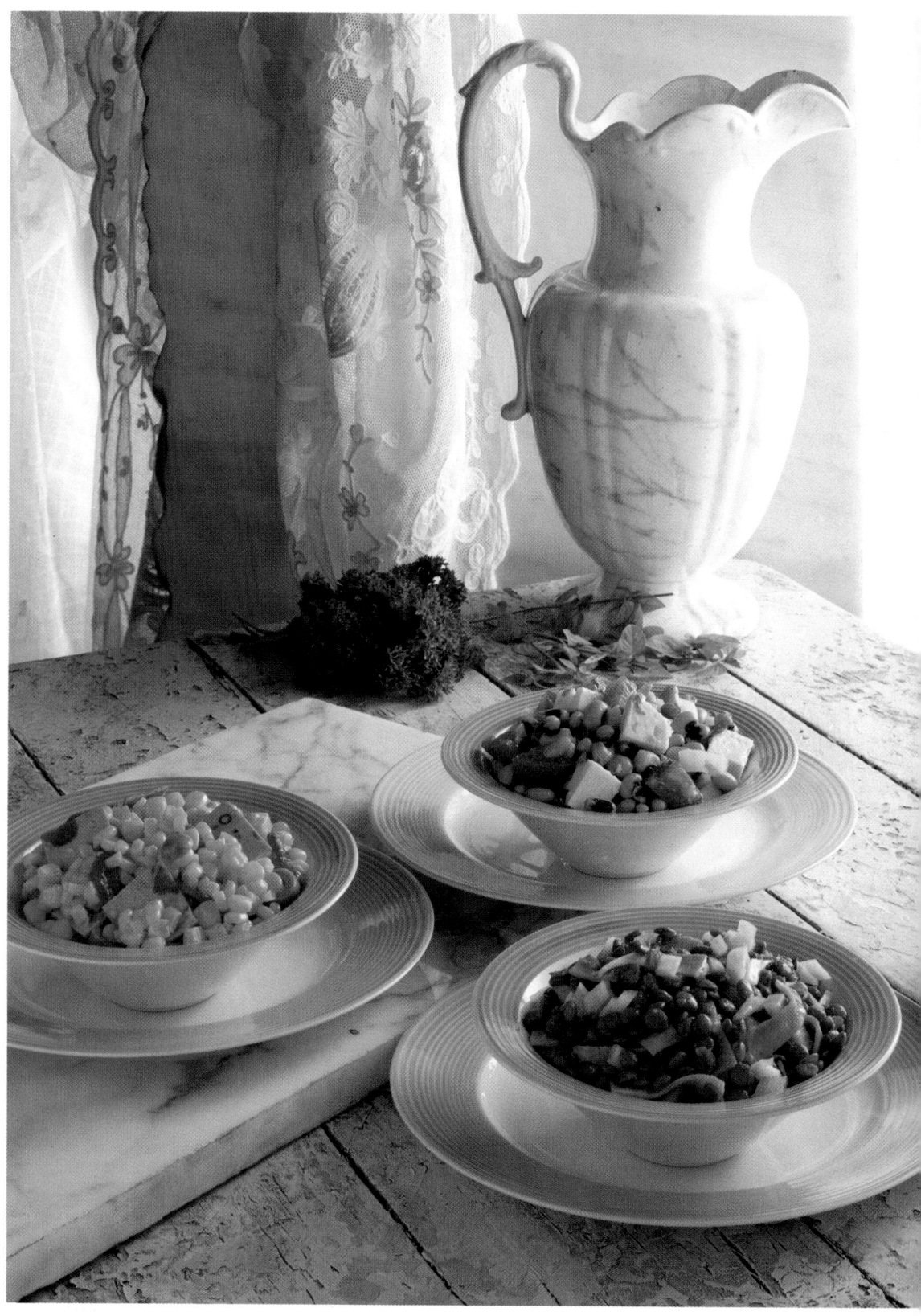

LEFT: SWEETCORN SALAD; TOP: GREEK BEAN
SALAD (P.48);

BOTTOM: VIENNESE LENTIL SALAD (P.47)

SWEETCORN SALAD

1 × 200 g (7 oz) can sweetcorn kernels, drained
4 tablespoons sliced, stoned green olives
1 tablespoon chopped, canned pimiento
25 g/1 oz Edam cheese, diced or cut into strips
4 tablespoons Apple juice dressing (page 58)

SERVES 4
Per serving: **Energy**   145 kcal/600 kJ
               Fat   11 g
               Fibre   3 g

Mix the sweetcorn with the olives, pimiento and cheese in a salad bowl.

Pour the dressing over the salad and toss to mix. Cover and chill for 10 minutes to allow the flavours to develop. Toss before serving.

COLOURFUL BEAN SALAD

450 g/1 lb green beans, topped and tailed
pinch of grated nutmeg
500 g/1¼ lb new potatoes, scrubbed and boiled
   in their skins
3–4 tomatoes, chopped or cut into wedges
1 medium onion, peeled and chopped
1½ tablespoons chopped fresh herbs (e.g.
   chives, parsley, thyme)
6 tablespoons Yogurt dressing (page 58)
freshly ground black pepper

SERVES 4–6
4 servings
Per serving: **Energy**   150 kcal/635 kJ
               Fat   2 g
               Fibre   7 g

6 servings
Per serving: **Energy**   100 kcal/420 kJ
               Fat   1 g
               Fibre   5 g

Steam the beans with the nutmeg for 10–12 minutes until just tender. Drain, rinse under cold water and transfer to a serving bowl. Add the potatoes and tomatoes and toss well. Scatter the onion and herbs on top. Pour the dressing over the bean salad, season and toss well to mix.

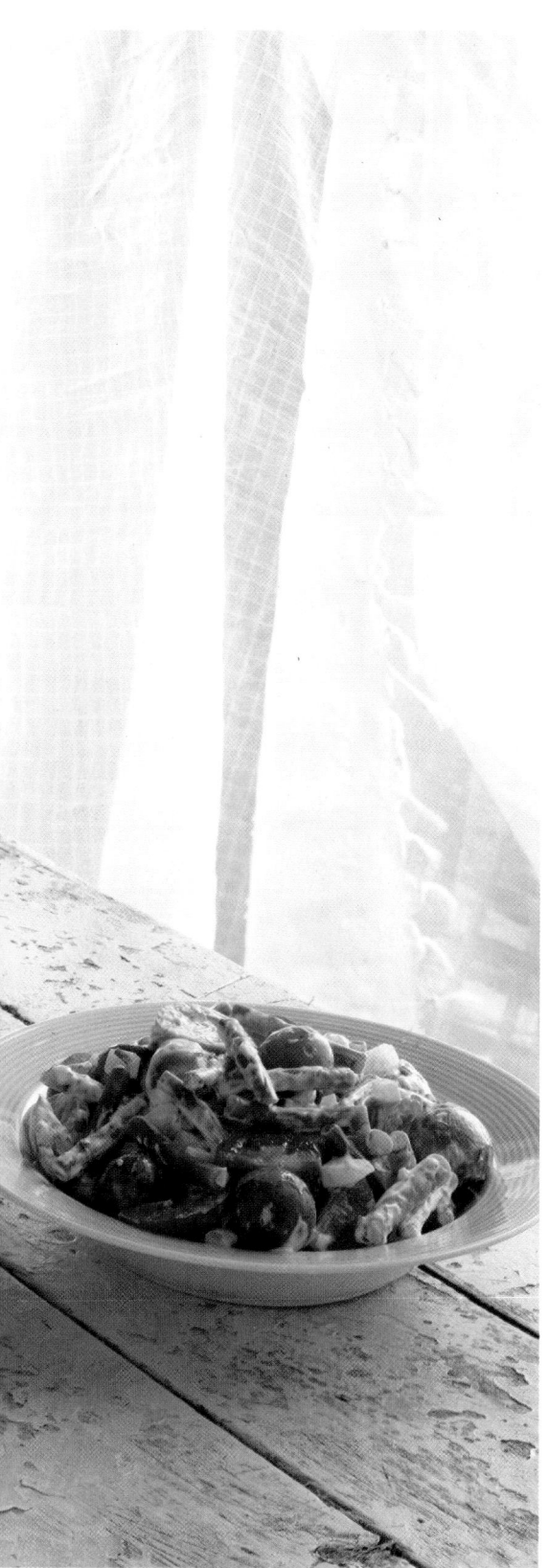

ABOVE: COLOURFUL BEAN SALAD

MINTED MELON AND STRAWBERRY COCKTAIL

1 small ripe honeydew or cantaloupe melon
100 g/4 oz strawberries, hulled and sliced
5 cm/2 inch piece cucumber, sliced and quartered
finely grated rind of 1 large orange
3–4 tablespoons orange juice
2 tablespoons chopped fresh mint
15 g/½ oz split blanched pistachio nuts or
  toasted almonds
½ small lettuce, shredded
TO GARNISH
4–6 mint sprigs

SERVES 4–6
4 servings
Per serving:	Energy	130 kcal/540 kJ
	Fat	10 g
	Fibre	4 g

6 servings
Per serving:	Energy	85 kcal/360 kJ
	Fat	7 g
	Fibre	3 g

Cut the melon into quarters, then remove the seeds and skin. Cut the flesh into 1 cm/½ inch cubes or scoop into balls. Place in a bowl with the strawberries and cucumber.

Mix the orange rind and juice with the mint and nuts, then pour on to the salad. Fold gently to mix.

Divide the lettuce equally between individual serving dishes or glasses. Spoon the salad on top, pouring in any orange juice from the bowl. Serve chilled, garnished with sprigs of mint.

VARIATION
If obtainable, ogen melons make an attractive variation. Cut them in half, discard the seeds and scoop out the flesh in balls. Serve the salad in the melon shells.

AUTUMN SLAW

225 g/8 oz red cabbage, shredded
2 dessert apples, unpeeled, cored and sliced
50 g/2 oz raisins

25 g/1 oz unsalted peanuts
4 celery sticks, chopped
4–5 tablespoons Apple juice dressing (page 58)

SERVES 4–6
4 servings
Per serving:	Energy	170 kcal/714 kJ
	Fat	10 g
	Fibre	4 g

6 servings
Per serving:	Energy	110 kcal/470 kJ
	Fat	7 g
	Fibre	3 g

Put the cabbage, apples, raisins, peanuts and celery in a bowl. Pour the dressing over the salad and toss.

SESAME SPINACH SALAD

450 g/1 lb spinach
2 tablespoons sesame seeds
2 teaspoons sesame oil
1 teaspoon cider vinegar
freshly ground black pepper

SERVES 4
Per serving:	Energy	100 kcal/420 kJ
	Fat	7 g
	Fibre	8 g

Cook the spinach in a little boiling water for 3 minutes. Drain the spinach, pressing to extract all excess moisture.

Heat the sesame seeds in a frying pan, then grind them in a mortar with a pestle. Add the oil and vinegar to the ground sesame seeds and mix well. Season with black pepper to taste.

Cut the spinach into 4 cm/1½ inch lengths. Add the sesame seed mixture and toss to coat the spinach. Serve in a shallow dish.

CARROT SALAD

225 g/8 oz endive
350 g/12 oz carrots, scrubbed and finely grated
2 medium oranges, peeled and segmented
75 g/3 oz stoned dates
2 tablespoons lemon juice
TO GARNISH
50 g/2 oz watercress

SERVES 4
Per serving: **Energy** 90 kcal/385 kJ
Fat negligible
Fibre 7 g

Arrange the endive around the base and sides of a salad bowl. Combine the remaining ingredients and spoon over the endive. Garnish with watercress.

NUTTY CAULIFLOWER SALAD

1 cauliflower, broken into florets
50 g/2 oz hazelnuts, chopped
50 g/2 oz Camembert cheese, diced
75 g/3 oz watercress
4 tablespoons Apple juice dressing (page 58)

SERVES 4
Per serving: **Energy** 160 kcal/680 kJ
Fat 15 g
Fibre 2 g

Steam the cauliflower until just tender but still crisp. Drain well and cool.

Mix the cauliflower, nuts, cheese and watercress in a salad bowl. Pour the dressing over the salad ingredients and toss gently. Serve lightly chilled.

CHESTNUT SALAD

225 g/8 oz whole chestnuts, skinned (page 36)
175 g/6 oz Brussels sprouts, grated
2 celery sticks, diced
1 large orange, peeled and segmented
3 tablespoons Apple juice dressing (page 58)

SERVES 4
Per serving: **Energy** 170 kcal/715 kJ
Fat 7 g
Fibre 7 g

Put the chestnuts into a saucepan with sufficient water to cover. Bring to the boil, then simmer for about 15 minutes or until the chestnuts are cooked. Drain thoroughly and leave to cool.

Chop the chestnuts and mix with the remaining ingredients. This salad is good served with cold turkey.

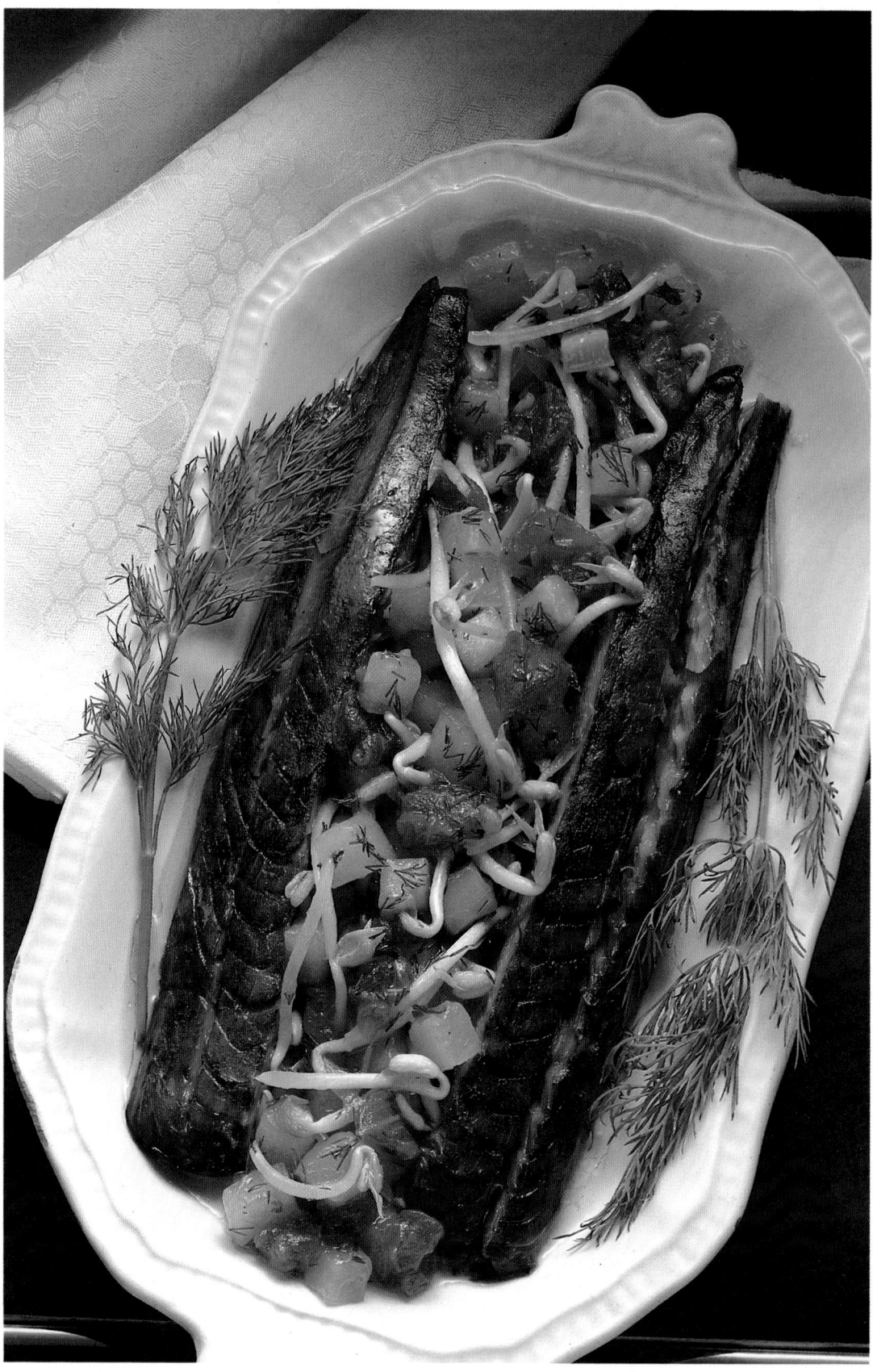

CHICORY AND POTATO SALAD

2 medium heads chicory
1 teaspoon lemon juice
2 tablespoons plain unsweetened yogurt
freshly ground black pepper
450 g/1 lb new potatoes, scrubbed, steamed in
    their skins, and diced
1 × 175 g (6 oz) can tuna fish, drained and
    wiped
225 g/8 oz green beans, sliced and cooked
4 tomatoes, quartered

20 black olives
TO GARNISH
chopped chives

SERVES 4
Per serving: **Energy** 185 kcal/770 kJ
              Fat 11 g
              Fibre 5 g

Separate the chicory leaves and arrange around the edge of a serving plate. Stir the lemon juice into the yogurt and season with pepper. Mix with the diced potatoes and spoon into the middle of the serving plate. Mix together the tuna, beans, tomatoes and olives and arrange around the edge of the potatoes.

Garnish the salad with chopped fresh chives.

SMOKED MACKEREL SALAD

6 tablespoons bean-sprouts
½ cucumber, unpeeled and cut into 5 mm/¼
    inch dice
4 firm tomatoes
2 tablespoons lemon juice
4 small smoked mackerel fillets

SERVES 4
Per serving: **Energy** 350 kcal/1465 kJ
              Fat 24 g
              Fibre 2 g

Rinse the bean-sprouts in cold water, drain thoroughly and chill in the refrigerator until ready to serve.

Combine the bean-sprouts with the cucumber and tomatoes and toss lightly in the lemon juice.

Arrange the fillets of fish on individual plates and serve with the salad.

RED BEAN SALAD

120 g/4½ oz red beans, soaked overnight in
    cold water
600 ml/1 pint water
4 tablespoons Sesame dressing (page 58)
TO GARNISH
1 tablespoon chopped fresh parsley

SERVES 4
Per serving: **Energy** 130 kcal/555 kJ
              Fat 5 g
              Fibre 8 g

Drain the beans and put into a saucepan with the water. Bring to the boil and boil rapidly for 10 minutes. Then reduce the heat and simmer for about 45 minutes until tender, adding further water if necessary. Drain carefully and toss the beans with the Sesame dressing. Garnish the dish with chopped parsley.

OPPOSITE: SMOKED MACKEREL SALAD

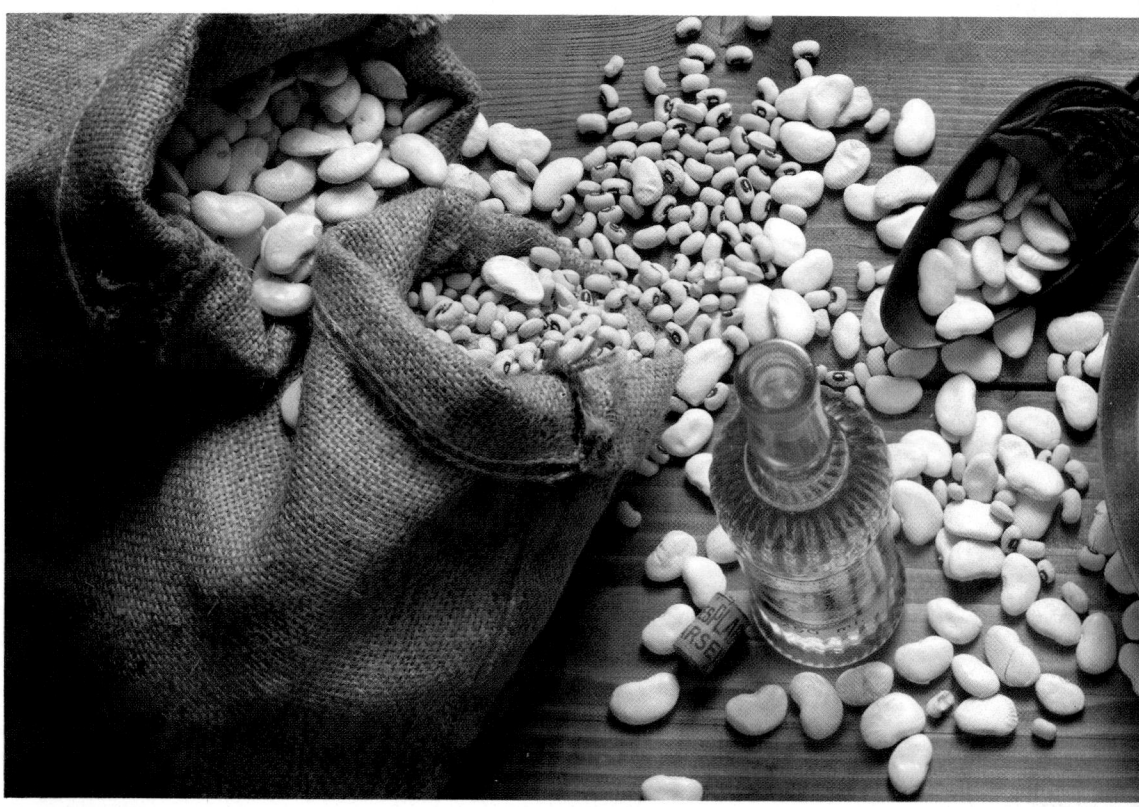

WHITE BEAN SALAD

WHITE BEAN SALAD

*225 g/8 oz dried white beans (mixture of
  haricot, butter and black-eye beans), soaked
  overnight in cold water*
600 ml/1 pint water
1 onion, finely chopped
1 bay leaf
freshly ground black pepper
2 tablespoons lemon juice
grated rind of 1 small lemon
1 tablespoon capers

2 gherkins, sliced
2 tablespoons chopped fresh parsley
3 tablespoons Apple juice dressing (page 58)
2 hard-boiled eggs, cut into wedges
8 black olives

SERVES 6 as an hors d'oeuvre
Per serving: Energy 195 kcal/810 kJ
              Fat   8 g
              Fibre 10 g

Drain the beans and place in a saucepan with the water. Bring to the boil and boil rapidly for 10 minutes. Then add the onion and bay leaf with pepper to taste. Cover the pan and simmer for 45 minutes – 1 hour or until the beans are tender. Drain the beans and leave to cool thoroughly.

Mix the lemon juice and rind, capers, gherkins, parsley with the dressing. Pour half the dressing over the beans and leave to marinate for at least 30 minutes. Discard the bay leaf. Turn the beans into a serving dish and arrange the hard-boiled eggs and olives on the top. Add the remaining dressing and serve.

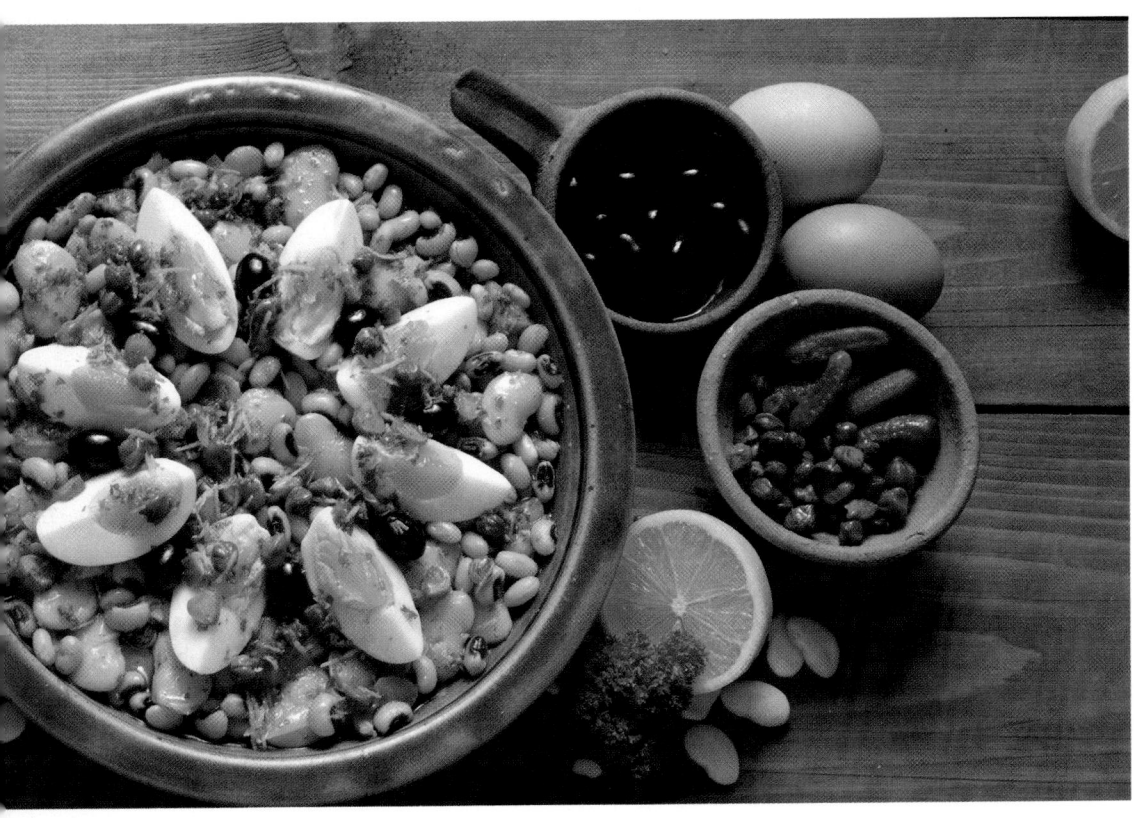

BROAD BEAN SALAD

225 g/8 oz small raw broad beans, shelled
   weight
½ medium cucumber, unpeeled and diced
2 medium oranges, peeled and sliced
6 radishes, sliced
1 tablespoon chopped fresh mint
2–3 tablespoons Apple juice dressing (page 58)

SERVES 4
Per serving: **Energy** 105 kcal/435 kJ
              Fat   6 g
              Fibre   4 g

Mix the ingredients together. Serve with
crusty wholemeal rolls.

SPINACH AND WALNUT SALAD

175 g/6 oz spinach, washed and drained
40 g/1½ oz walnuts, chopped
2 shallots, finely chopped
2–3 tablespoons Apple juice dressing (page 58)

SERVES 4
Per serving: **Energy** 100 kcal/430 kJ
              Fat   9 g
              Fibre   3 g

Tear the well drained spinach into small
pieces and place with the walnuts and
shallots in a salad bowl. Pour the dressing
over the salad and toss well.

Picnics & Barbecues

GRAPEFRUIT TUNA PÂTÉ

*1 × 200 g (7 oz) can tuna fish, drained and
wiped
grated rind of 1 grapefruit
segments of 1 grapefruit*

*75 g/3 oz fresh wholemeal breadcrumbs
2 teaspoons grated onion
1 egg, beaten
freshly ground black pepper*

SERVES 4–6
4 servings
Per serving: Energy 210 kcal/880 kJ
            Fat 13 g
            Fibre 2 g

6 servings
Per serving: Energy 140 kcal/585 kJ
            Fat 9 g
            Fibre 1 g

Mash the tuna until smooth, then mix in the remaining ingredients with pepper to taste. Spoon into a greased 450 g (1 lb) loaf tin and smooth the top.

Bake in a preheated moderate oven (180°C, 350°F, Gas Mark 4) for 40 minutes. Cool in the tin, then turn out on to a serving plate. Serve chilled.

TUNA PÂTÉ

*1 × 200 g (7 oz) can tuna fish, drained, wiped
and flaked
2 hard-boiled eggs, chopped
225 g/8 oz low-fat soft cheese or sieved cottage
cheese
2 tablespoons chopped fresh chives
2 tablespoons chopped fresh parsley
2 tablespoons brandy (optional)
freshly ground black pepper*

SERVES 4–6
4 servings
Per serving: Energy 255 kcal/1060 kJ
            Fat 16 g
            Fibre negligible
6 servings
Per serving: Energy 170 kcal/710 kJ
            Fat 11 g
            Fibre negligible

Put all the ingredients, with pepper to taste, in a bowl and beat until well combined. For a very smooth pâté, use a blender or food processor. Spoon into a small serving dish and chill before serving with wholemeal rolls.

MUSHROOM AND ALMOND PÂTÉ

1–2 tablespoons olive oil
225 g/8 oz mushrooms, chopped
2 spring onions, finely chopped
65 g/2½ oz blanched almonds, toasted
100 g/4 oz quark cheese
freshly ground black pepper
pinch of dried tarragon (optional)

SERVES 4
Per serving: **Energy** 175 kcal/730 kJ
Fat 16 g
Fibre 4 g

Heat the oil in a frying pan and cook the mushrooms and spring onions gently until soft. Put this mixture into a blender with the almonds and quark cheese. Season with pepper and tarragon if used. Blend until smooth. Pack into a plastic container, cover and refrigerate for at least 3 hours. Serve with wholemeal rolls.

STUFFED VINE LEAVES

225 g/8 oz fresh or preserved vine leaves
150 g/5 oz long-grain brown rice, soaked in
  cold water for 15 minutes, rinsed and drained
350 g/12 oz onions, diced
50 g/2 oz pine nuts
25 g/1 oz blanched flaked almonds
25 g/1 oz raisins
4 tablespoons chopped fresh mint
2 tablespoons chopped fresh parsley
3 tablespoons chopped dill or fennel (optional)

4 tablespoons olive oil
5 tablespoons lemon juice
freshly ground black pepper
1 egg white

SERVES 6
Per serving: **Energy** 310 kcal/1310 kJ
Fat 20 g
Fibre 5 g

These are ideal for picnics as they can be prepared the day before and are easily held in the hand to eat.

If using fresh vine leaves, blanch them in boiling water for 2 minutes. Drain and rinse in cold water. Remove any stalks.

Cover the bottom of a large saucepan with 3–4 vine leaves.

Mix together the rice, onions, nuts, raisins, herbs, oil and 3 tablespoons of the lemon juice. Season to taste with pepper. Bind with the egg white. Put a teaspoon of the stuffing near the base of a vine leaf at the stem end. Roll the stuffing into the shape of a cork and fold over the stem end of the vine leaf. Fold both edges of the leaf over towards the middle and roll up into a small sausage.

Pack the stuffed vine leaves into the saucepan, keeping the joined edges underneath. Sprinkle each layer with pepper. Pour the remaining lemon juice over the top. Cover with a small heatproof plate. Add sufficient hot water to half-fill the pan. Cover and cook very slowly for 50 minutes. Then remove one stuffed vine leaf and test: if it is slightly too crunchy, cook for a few more minutes. The age of the fresh vine leaves affects the cooking time. If necessary, add a little more water.

POTTED TURKEY

225 g/8 oz cooked turkey meat
2 tablespoons olive oil
1 medium onion, very finely chopped
1–2 garlic cloves, crushed
50 g/2 oz black olives, chopped
75 g/3 oz red pepper, diced
1 tablespoon dry sherry or port
about 5 tablespoons chicken stock
freshly ground black pepper
pinch of ground mace or ground nutmeg
pinch of dried mixed herbs (optional)

SERVES 4–6

4 servings

Per serving:	Energy	170 kcal/715 kJ
	Fat	10 g
	Fibre	1 g

6 servings

Per serving:	Energy	115 kcal/475 kJ
	Fat	7 g
	Fibre	1 g

Cooked chicken meat or game can also be 'potted' in this way. Potted turkey will keep for 2–3 days in the refrigerator but not longer as it does not contain any kind of preservative.

Mince the turkey meat finely twice. Heat the oil in a frying pan, add the onion and garlic and cook gently until soft and lightly coloured. Stir in the minced turkey, olives and red pepper followed by the sherry or port and sufficient stock just to moisten. Season to taste with pepper and mace or nutmeg and add the herbs if used. Press the mixture into a plastic container and level the top. Chill until firm.

POTTED SALMON

1 × 200 g (7 oz) can salmon, drained and wiped
1 × 225 g (8 oz) carton cottage cheese with
   chives
100 g/4 oz frozen peas, cooked
2 tablespoons plain unsweetened yogurt
1 teaspoon Worcestershire sauce
freshly ground black pepper

SERVES 6–8

6 servings

Per serving:	Energy	100 kcal/410 kJ
	Fat	4 g
	Fibre	2 g

8 servings

Per serving:	Energy	75 kcal/305 kJ
	Fat	3 g
	Fibre	1 g

Purée all the ingredients with pepper to taste in a blender until smooth. Spoon the mixture into a plastic container and smooth the top. Cover and chill for several hours or overnight if possible. Serve as a spread with wholemeal crispbreads or toast.

OPPOSITE: DEVILLED TURKEY KEBABS WITH
APRICOT PILAFF (P.72)

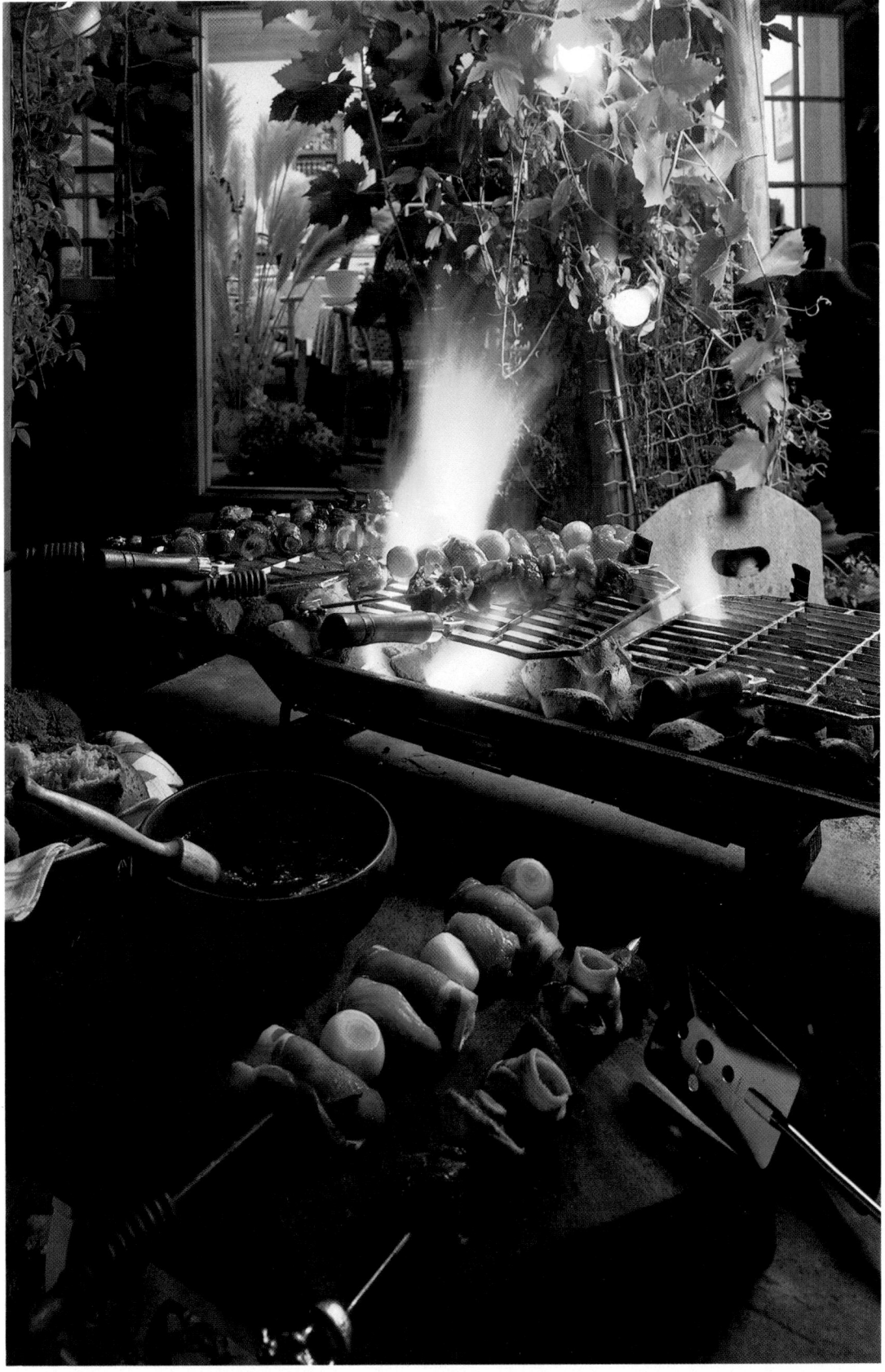

DEVILLED TURKEY KEBABS
WITH APRICOT PILAFF

PILAFF
1 tablespoon oil
1 medium onion, chopped
1 celery stick, sliced
225 g/8 oz long-grain brown rice
600 ml/1 pint chicken stock
50 g/2 oz raisins
75 g/3 oz dried apricots, roughly chopped
25 g/1 oz walnuts, roughly chopped

KEBABS
450 g/1 lb turkey meat, dark or white, cut into
2.5 cm/1 inch cubes
4 lean bacon rashers, rinded, halved and rolled
8 onion wedges, or 4 baby onions, halved
SAUCE
3 tablespoons canned unsweetened chestnut
purée
2 teaspoons Dijon mustard
1 garlic clove, crushed
2 tablespoons lemon juice

1 cinnamon stick
1 bay leaf
freshly ground black pepper

SERVES 4
Per serving: **Energy** 380 kcal/1585 kJ
Fat 12 g
Fibre 9 g

2 tablespoons orange juice
1 tablespoon corn oil
1 teaspoon Worcestershire sauce
grated rind of 1 orange
pinch of cayenne pepper
freshly ground black pepper

SERVES 4
Per serving: **Energy** 255 kcal/1075 kJ
Fat 9 g
Fibre 1 g

To make the pilaff, heat the oil in a pan. Add the onion and celery and cook gently for 5 minutes until golden brown. Add the rice and cook for 1 minute, stirring constantly. Pour on the stock, then add the raisins, apricots and walnuts. Bring to the boil stirring occasionally, then add the cinnamon, bay leaf and pepper to taste. Lower the heat, cover the pan and simmer for 30 minutes or until the rice is tender and all the stock has been absorbed. Remove the cinnamon and bay leaf.

Thread the turkey cubes on to 4 long skewers alternating with the bacon rolls and onions. Put the sauce ingredients in a pan and bring just to the boil. Remove quickly from the heat and brush the sauce all over the kebabs.

Cook on a hot barbecue or under a preheated moderate grill for 8–10 minutes on each side or until cooked through. Brush at least once more with the sauce during cooking.

Spoon the pilaff into a warmed shallow serving dish and arrange the kebabs on top. Serve immediately. *Illustrated on p. 71.*

COURGETTE KEBABS

2 courgettes, thickly sliced
200 g/7 oz small button mushrooms
3 tablespoons lemon juice
100 g/4 oz lean bacon, rinded, halved and
  rolled
200 g/7 oz turkey liver, cubed
freshly ground black pepper
ground paprika

chopped fresh basil
olive oil

SERVES 4
Per serving: **Energy** 150 kcal/630 kJ
Fat 9 g
Fibre 2 g

Sprinkle the courgettes and mushrooms with the lemon juice. Thread the courgettes, mushrooms, bacon rolls and turkey liver alternately on 4 long wooden skewers. Season with pepper, paprika and basil and brush lightly with oil.

Cook, over a barbecue or under a preheated hot grill, for about 10 minutes, turning occasionally until brown and crisp.

Season the courgettes lightly with pepper and serve immediately with wholemeal toast.

FRUIT KEBABS

1 green apple, unpeeled, cored and sliced thickly
1 red apple, unpeeled, cored and sliced thickly
2 bananas, peeled and sliced thickly
lemon juice
2 large oranges, peeled and segmented
12 black grapes
50 g/2 oz Edam cheese, cubed
mint sprigs (optional)

SERVES 4
Per serving: Energy 120 kcal/495 kJ
Fat 3 g
Fibre 3 g

Brush the apple and banana slices with a little lemon juice to prevent discolouring. Thread the apples, bananas, oranges, grapes and cheese alternately on 4 skewers. Cook on a barbecue or under a pre-heated hot grill until heated through. If cooking over charcoal, throw a few sprigs of mint on the coals during cooking to give the fruit a minted flavour.

Serve the kebabs hot.

BACON POTATOES

4 firm, even-sized potatoes
1 tablespoon olive oil
freshly ground black pepper
100 g/4 oz lean bacon, rinded, grilled until
  crisp, and chopped
3 medium tomatoes, diced
TO GARNISH
chopped fresh chives
plain unsweetened yogurt

SERVES 4
Per serving: Energy 210 kcal/890 kJ
Fat 4 g
Fibre 5 g

Scrub the potatoes well, and dry. Prick with a fork, brush with oil and sprinkle with pepper. Wrap each separately in a piece of aluminium foil. Place over hot coals or directly on the coals and cook for about 45 minutes–1 hour. Turn occasionally while cooking.

Remove from the foil and slice off the tops. Scoop out the soft potato and place in a bowl. Add the chopped bacon, tomatoes and pepper, mix well and pile back into the skins. Wrap the foil around the potatoes again, and reheat for about 15 minutes.

Top each potato with chives and yogurt.

Light Meals & Snacks

STUFFED ARTICHOKES

Cut the thick stems from the artichokes and trim the leaves with a pair of kitchen scissors. Place the artichokes in a large saucepan of boiling water, cover and simmer gently for 45 minutes. The artichokes are cooked when a leaf can be pulled out easily. Place the artichokes upside down in a colander and leave to drain.

Remove the choke by cutting carefully with a sharp knife and scooping out with a spoon.

Fill the artichokes, using one of the following four recipes for stuffings.

CAULIFLOWER STUFFING

175 g/6 oz cauliflower florets
25 g/1 oz mushrooms, chopped
1 tablespoon diced lean bacon
1 tablespoon tomato purée
1 tablespoon chicken stock
freshly ground black pepper
25 g/1 oz Edam cheese, grated

MAKES stuffing for 2 artichokes
Per serving: Energy 120 kcal/495 kJ
              Fat   4 g
              Fibre 4 g
(includes the artichoke)

Combine the cauliflower, mushrooms and bacon. Mix in the tomato purée and stock. Season with pepper. Place in a casserole in a preheated moderate oven (180°C, 350°F, Gas Mark 4) for 45 minutes. Spoon into the artichokes and sprinkle over the cheese. Place under a preheated grill until the cheese is melted and golden brown.

Serve the artichokes immediately. *Illustrated on p. 75.*

OPPOSITE: ARTICHOKES WITH VARIOUS STUFFINGS. FROM LEFT: CHICKEN (P.76), VEGETARIAN (P.76), CAULIFLOWER (ABOVE) AND PRAWN (P.76)

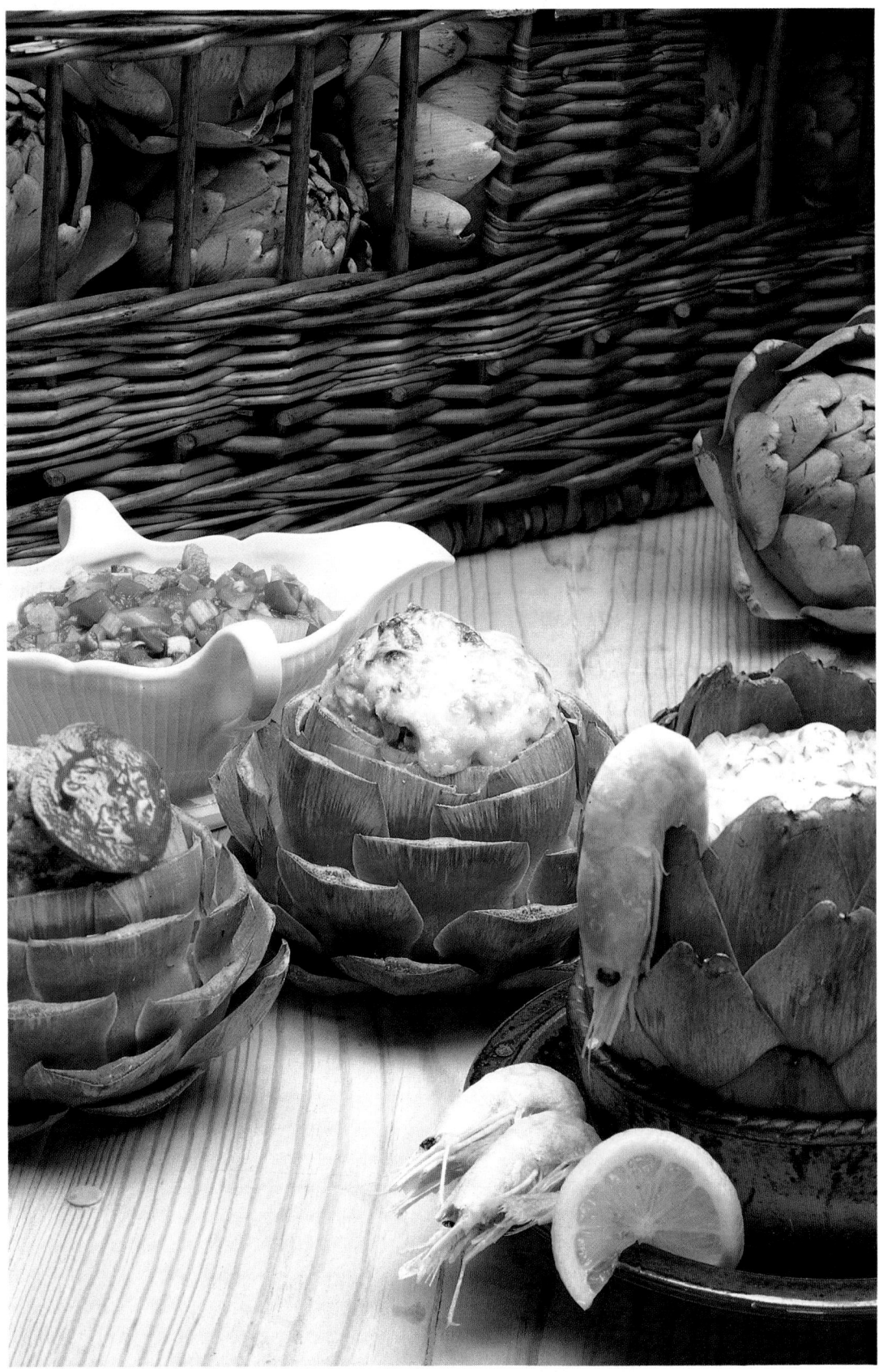

VEGETARIAN STUFFING

1 tablespoon olive oil
½ green pepper, cored, seeded and diced
1 celery stick, chopped
1 tablespoon finely chopped onion
50 g / 2 oz mushrooms, chopped
150 ml / ¼ pint tomato juice
freshly ground black pepper

MAKES stuffing for 2 artichokes
Per serving: Energy 125 kcal / 530 kJ
Fat 8 g
Fibre 3 g
(includes the artichoke)

Heat the oil and fry the pepper, celery, onion and mushrooms. Add the tomato juice and season with pepper. Simmer for 30 minutes. Spoon into the artichokes. Serve hot or cold. *Illustrated on p. 75.*

PRAWN STUFFING

50 g / 2 oz peeled fresh or frozen prawns
150 ml / ¼ pint plain unsweetened yogurt
1 tablespoon chopped chives
1 teaspoon capers
½ teaspoon dried tarragon
TO GARNISH
2 unshelled prawns

MAKES stuffing for 2 artichokes
Per serving: Energy 110 kcal / 460 kJ
Fat 4 g
Fibre 2 g
(includes the artichoke)

Combine all the ingredients and divide between the artichokes. Garnish with the unshelled prawns. *Illustrated on p. 75.*

CHICKEN STUFFING

100 g / 4 oz cooked chicken, diced
50 g / 2 oz cooked green peas
3 tablespoons plain unsweetened yogurt
freshly ground black pepper
TO GARNISH
2 tomatoes, sliced

MAKES stuffing for 2 artichokes
Per serving: Energy 140 kcal / 595 kJ
Fat 4 g
Fibre 4 g
(includes the artichoke)

Combine all the ingredients and divide between the artichokes. Garnish with the tomato slices. *Illustrated on p. 75.*

STUFFED ONIONS

4 large Spanish onions, boiled in their skins for
   45 minutes
1 celery stick, diced
1 medium cooking apple, peeled, cored and diced
100 g/4 oz fresh wholemeal breadcrumbs
1 tablespoon chopped fresh parsley
1 teaspoon chopped fresh thyme
1 large tomato, chopped

1 garlic clove, crushed
freshly ground black pepper
175 ml/6 fl oz chicken stock

SERVES 4
Per serving: **Energy** 85 kcal/360 kJ
                Fat 1 g
                Fibre 4 g

Peel and cool the onions. Scoop out part of the centres and chop finely. Mix the chopped onion with the remaining ingredients, except for the stock. Pack this mixture into the onion cases and arrange these in a shallow ovenproof dish. Pour the stock over the stuffed onions. Cook in a preheated moderate oven (160°C, 325°F, Gas Mark 3) for about 1 hour. The time taken depends on the size of the onions.

PRUNE-STUFFED TOMATOES

4 large tomatoes
100 g/4 oz quark cheese
2 teaspoons plain unsweetened yogurt
10 cooked prunes, stoned and chopped
freshly ground black pepper
4 walnut halves

SERVES 4
Per serving: **Energy** 65 kcal/275 kJ
                Fat 1 g
                Fibre 4 g

Cut a lid from the top of each tomato and reserve. Scoop out the insides of the tomatoes, then place them upside-down on absorbent kitchen paper to drain.

Beat the cheese and yogurt together, then mix in the prunes. Season the insides of the tomatoes with pepper and fill with the prune mixture. Place a walnut half on top of each, then add the tomato lids. Chill lightly before serving.

SAVOURY BAKED APPLES

4 large cooking apples
75 g/3 oz cooked chicken, finely chopped
75 g/3 oz cooked long-grain brown rice
25 g/1 oz red pepper, diced
½ teaspoon coriander
1 teaspoon tomato purée
1 teaspoon chopped fresh tarragon (optional)
175 ml/6 fl oz chicken stock

SERVES 4
Per serving: **Energy** 130 kcal/545 kJ
                Fat 1 g
                Fibre 4 g

Run the tip of a sharp knife around each apple. Remove the cores and enlarge the central holes slightly. Mix the chicken, rice, red pepper, coriander, tomato purée and tarragon, if used, together thoroughly. Stuff the mixture into the apple cavities. Put each apple into an individual ovenproof dish and pour some chicken stock into each. Bake in a moderate oven (180°C, 350°F, Gas Mark 4) for about 40 minutes.

FISH WITH CRUNCHY TOPPING

450 g / 1 lb haddock fillets
150 g / 5 oz walnuts, milled
75 g / 3 oz wholemeal breadcrumbs
3 tablespoons milled parsley
1 tablespoon olive oil
3 tablespoons lemon juice
1–2 garlic cloves, crushed

SERVES 4
Per serving: **Energy** 375 kcal / 1580 kJ
Fat 24 g
Fibre 4 g

Arrange the fish in a lightly oiled shallow ovenproof dish. Mix the remaining ingredients to a paste and spread this evenly over the fish, pressing it down firmly. Bake in a preheated moderate oven (180°C, 350°F, Gas Mark 4) for 15–20 minutes.

Remove the fish to a warmed serving dish and serve with a green salad.

MULLET IN A PARCEL

2 red mullet
freshly ground black pepper
75 g / 3 oz rolled oats
10 g / ½ oz bran
225 g / 8 oz courgettes, sliced
75 g / 3 oz mushrooms, thinly sliced
1 garlic clove, crushed
1 tablespoon lemon juice
1 tablespoon apple juice
pinch dried fennel
TO GARNISH
fresh fennel sprigs
lemon slices

SERVES 2
Per serving: **Energy** 260 kcal / 1080 kJ
Fat 7 g
Fibre 7 g

Slit each mullet along the belly, snip off the fins and wash the fish thoroughly in cold running water, removing the gut. Keep the fish whole. Place on a piece of foil and season with pepper.

Toast the rolled oats in a hot frying pan. Combine with the bran and remaining ingredients and divide this mixture around each fish. Cook in a preheated moderately hot oven (190°C, 375°F, Gas Mark 5) for 30 minutes.

To serve the fish, open the foil parcel. Garnish with fennel and lemon slices.

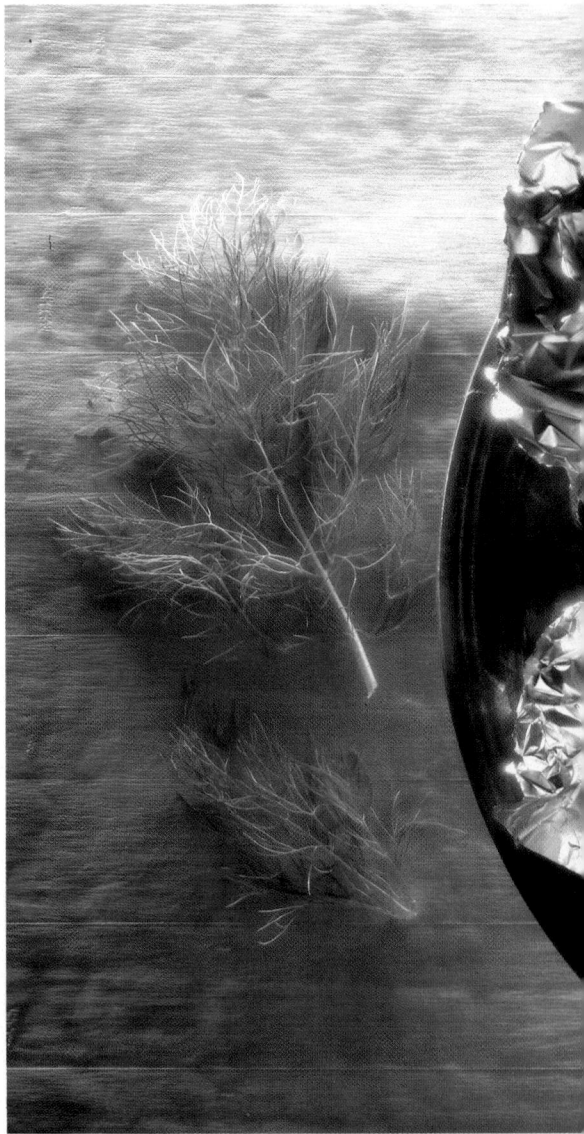

KOHLRABI CASSEROLE

5–6 kohlrabi, peeled, finely sliced or chopped
2 teaspoons olive oil
1 sprig parsley, coarsely chopped
100 g/4 oz Camembert cheese, cubed
50 g/2 oz lean bacon, rinded, grilled and diced
300 ml/½ pint skimmed milk, warmed
grated nutmeg

SERVES 4
Per serving: **Energy** 170 kcal/720 kJ
           Fat 10 g
           Fibre 1 g

Place the kohlrabi in a casserole and sprinkle with the oil. Add the parsley, cheese, bacon, milk and nutmeg to taste. Mix well and cook in a preheated moderately hot oven (200°C, 400°F, Gas Mark 6) for 20–30 minutes. *Illustrated on p. 38.*

MULLET IN A PARCEL

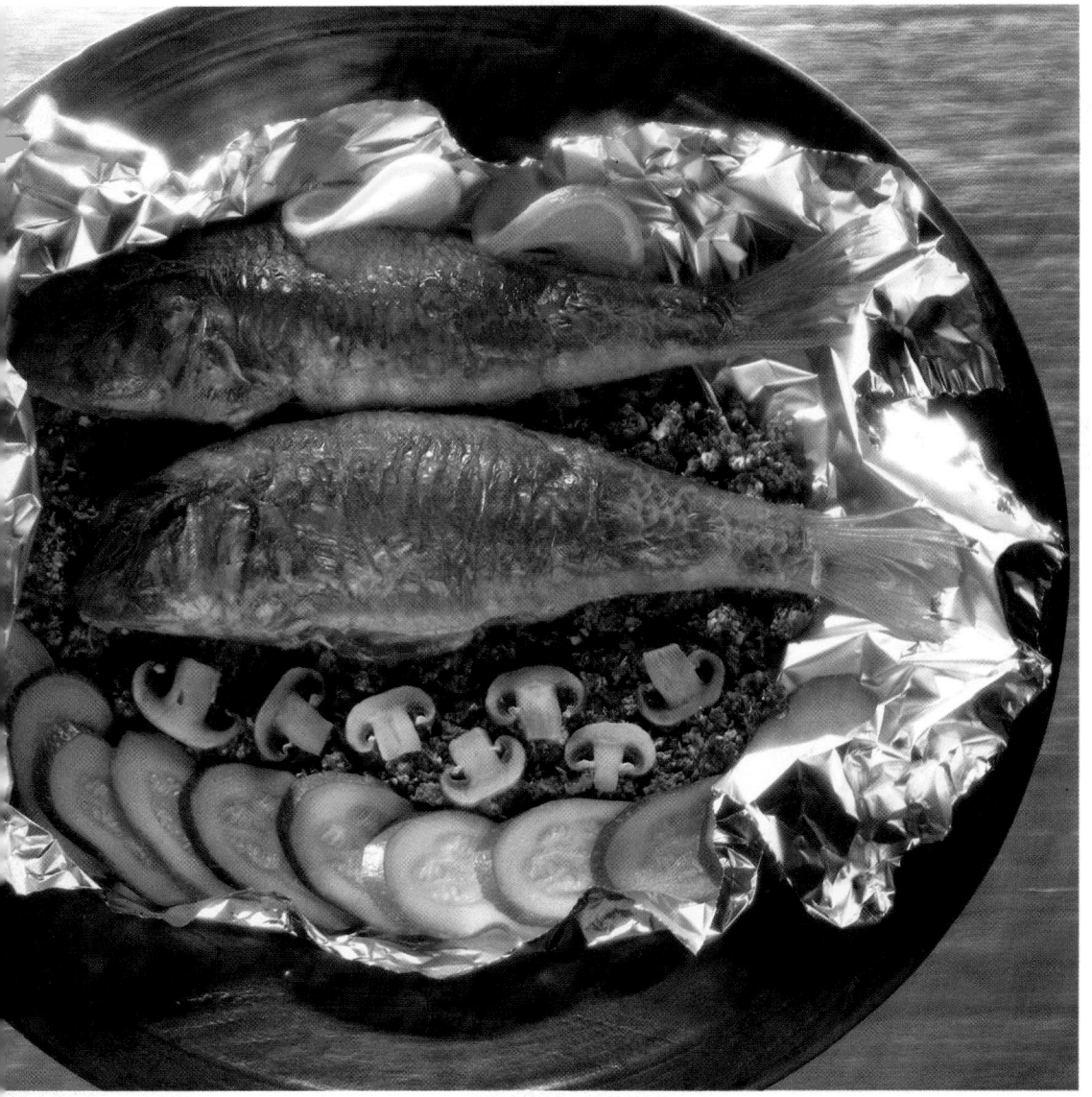

VEGETABLE RISOTTO

1 tablespoon olive oil
1 medium onion, chopped
1 garlic clove, crushed
225 g/8 oz long-grain brown rice
5 tomatoes, quartered
600 ml/1 pint chicken stock
freshly ground black pepper
finely grated rind of ½ lemon
2 sprigs fresh rosemary, chopped or 1 teaspoon
    dried rosemary

75 g/3 oz frozen or canned sweetcorn
75 g/3 oz frozen peas
50 g/2 oz green olives, sliced
TO GARNISH
lemon slices

SERVES 4
Per serving: Energy 285 kcal/1195 kJ
            Fat   7 g
            Fibre 7 g

Heat the oil in a pan and cook the onion and garlic for 3 minutes. Add the rice and cook for a further 2 minutes.

Add the tomatoes, stock, pepper, lemon rind and rosemary. Bring to the boil, cover and simmer for 15 minutes. Add the sweetcorn and peas and cook gently for a further 10 minutes or until the rice is cooked and the liquid absorbed. Stir in the olives and garnish with lemon slices.

BAKED CELERY

1 head celery, scrubbed and chopped
25 g/1 oz margarine
25 g/1 oz wholemeal flour
150 ml/¼ pint skimmed milk
50 g/2 oz Edam cheese, grated
25 g/1 oz wholemeal breadcrumbs

SERVES 4
Per serving: Energy 140 kcal/585 kJ
            Fat   8 g
            Fibre 3 g

Cook the celery in a little boiling water for 10–15 minutes. Drain well, retaining 150 ml/¼ pint of the liquor. Melt the margarine in a small pan, blend in the flour and cook over a low heat for 3 minutes. Add the celery liquor and the skimmed milk, stirring continuously until smooth. Add half the cheese and stir to blend. Fill an ovenproof dish with alternate layers of celery and sauce. Sprinkle with the remaining cheese mixed with the breadcrumbs. Bake in a preheated moderately hot oven (190°C, 375°F, Gas Mark 5) oven until lightly browned.

TUNA-STUFFED AUBERGINES

2 large aubergines
1 tablespoon olive oil
1 medium onion, chopped
1 × 425 g (15 oz) can tomatoes, drained
2 tablespoons tomato purée
1 garlic clove, crushed
1 teaspoon mixed dried herbs
freshly ground black pepper

1 × 225 g (8 oz) can tuna fish, drained and
    wiped
75 g/3 oz Edam cheese, grated

SERVES 4
Per serving: Energy 305 kcal/1275 kJ
            Fat   23 g
            Fibre 4 g

Cut the aubergines lengthways in half. Using a grapefruit knife, carefully remove the inside flesh and chop roughly.

Heat the oil in a pan and fry the onion until brown. Add the tomatoes, tomato purée, garlic, aubergine flesh, herbs and pepper. Bring to the boil, then simmer for 15–20 minutes. Flake the tuna and stir into the mixture.

Pile into the aubergine shells and sprinkle with grated cheese. Cover and bake in a preheated moderately hot oven (190°C, 375°F, Gas Mark 5) for 30–35 minutes until golden brown.

PEANUT-STUFFED CHICKEN BREASTS

4 × 225 g (8 oz) boneless chicken breasts
3 tablespoons Crunchy peanut butter (page 120)

SERVES 4
Per serving: Energy 385 kcal/1620 kJ
Fat 12 g
Fibre 2 g

Lay the chicken breasts between two pieces of damp greaseproof paper and beat with a rolling pin until they are thin enough to stuff and roll.

Spread evenly with the peanut butter. Roll up and secure with a wooden cocktail stick or tie with cotton. Place in a grill pan and cook under a preheated moderate grill for about 5 minutes. Turn over to brown the other sides.

Remove the cotton if used, before serving the chicken breasts with a green salad.

LEEK AND BACON GRATIN

8 large leeks, white and pale green part washed
and sliced into 5 cm/2 inch lengths
2 large carrots, scrubbed and sliced into 5 cm/2
inch lengths
4 rashers lean bacon
SAUCE
25 g/1 oz margarine
25 g/1 oz wholemeal flour
300 ml/½ pint skimmed milk
freshly ground black pepper

grated nutmeg
TO FINISH
50 g/2 oz Edam cheese, grated
75 g/3 oz fresh wholemeal breadcrumbs

SERVES 4
Per serving: Energy 260 kcal/1105 kJ
Fat 10 g
Fibre 8 g

Cook the sliced leeks and carrots in boiling water to cover for 10–15 minutes or until tender. Drain, reserving the liquid, and turn into a flameproof casserole.

Meanwhile prepare the sauce. Melt the margarine in a pan, stir in the flour and cook for 2–3 minutes, stirring constantly. Remove the pan from the heat and gradually add the milk and 150 ml/¼ pint of the liquid from the vegetables, stirring constantly. Return the pan to the heat. Bring to the boil slowly, stirring all the time. Lower the heat, season with pepper and nutmeg to taste and simmer gently until the sauce thickens.

Grill the bacon rashers, arrange on top of the leeks and carrots and cover with the sauce. Sprinkle thickly with the mixed cheese and breadcrumbs. Place the dish under a preheated hot grill until the surface is golden-brown and crisp. Serve the gratin immediately.

STUFFED GREEN PANCAKES

PANCAKES
100 g / 4 oz spinach, washed and drained
100 g / 4 oz wholemeal flour
1 egg
150 ml / ¼ pint skimmed milk
FILLING
450 g / 1 oz spinach, washed and drained
freshly ground black pepper

100 g / 4 oz low-fat soft cheese
1 tablespoon chopped chives

SERVES 4
Per serving: **Energy** 175 kcal / 730 kJ
       Fat 4 g
       Fibre 10 g

Poach the spinach with a little water until the leaves collapse and turn bright green. Place in a blender and make a thin purée.

Place the flour in a bowl. Beat in the egg and milk, then the spinach purée. Allow the batter to stand for 20 minutes before using.

Meanwhile, make the filling. Steam the spinach for about 6 minutes. When cool enough to handle, squeeze out as much moisture as possible in the hands, then chop finely. Season with pepper. Mix together the cheese and chives.

Heat a non-stick frying pan and use the batter to make 8 small pancakes. Divide the spinach between the pancakes and put about a teaspoonful of the cheese mixture at each end. Roll up the pancakes.

HERB GNOCCHI

350 g / 12 oz spinach, washed and drained
75 g / 3 oz watercress, washed and drained
50 g / 2 oz parsley, washed and drained
1 tablespoon chopped chervil
1 tablespoon chopped tarragon
1 tablespoon chopped dill
175 g / 6 oz low-fat soft cheese
freshly ground black pepper

2 eggs, beaten
2½ tablespoons wholemeal flour
25 g / 1 oz freshly grated Parmesan cheese

SERVES 4
Per serving: **Energy** 185 kcal / 770 kJ
       Fat 7 g
       Fibre 9 g

Start the day before. Steam the spinach, watercress and parsley for 6 minutes, then drain. When cool enough to handle, squeeze out as much moisture as possible in the hands, then chop finely. Add the chopped herbs and stir the purée in a saucepan over a low heat for several minutes, to dry it out.

Beat the soft cheese to a smooth consistency, and add to the purée with pepper. Take the pan off the heat. Stir the beaten eggs into the mixture. Finally, stir in the flour and beat until smooth. Pour into a shallow dish and leave to cool. Place in the refrigerator, uncovered, and leave overnight. (It can be left for 2 days if preferred.)

After chilling, the mixture should have become firm enough to handle; if not, this is because the green purée was too moist. If it is, stir in a little extra flour – but not much, or the gnocchi will be heavy.

Have a large pan of water on the boil, and form the green mixture into egg-shaped gnocchi, using two teaspoons and rolling them very lightly on a floured board. Drop them in batches into the pan; do not crowd them. When they float to the surface, after 4–5 minutes, lift them out with a slotted spoon and drain on a cloth. Test one to make sure they are cooked through, then transfer to a hot serving dish while you cook the others. Sprinkle the gnocchi with the Parmesan cheese.

OPPOSITE, TOP: HERB GNOCCHI;

BOTTOM: GREEN PANCAKES

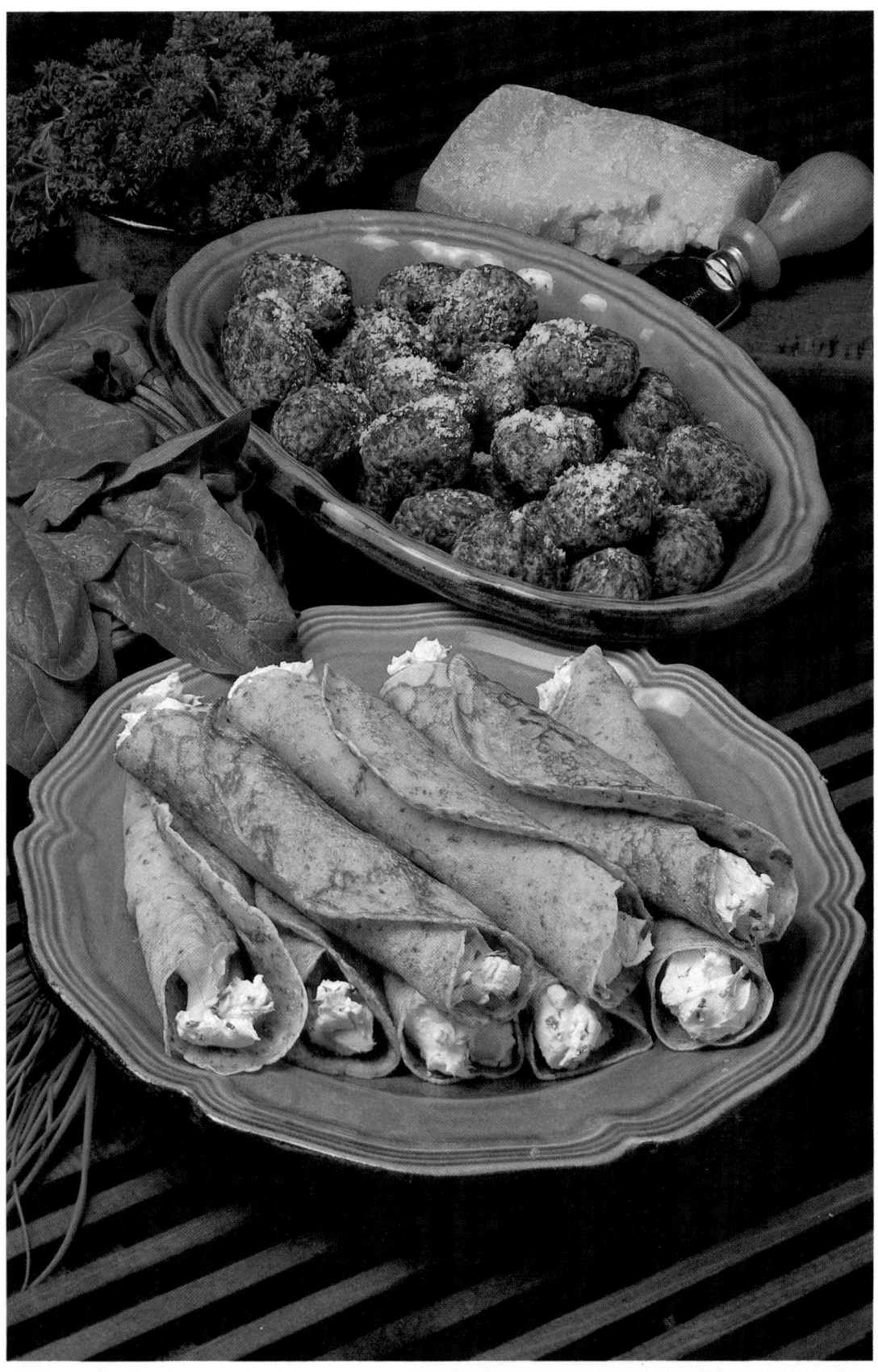

VEGETABLE CANNELLONI

8 wholemeal cannelloni tubes
2 × 400 g (14 oz) cans tomatoes
100 g/4 oz wholemeal breadcrumbs
50 g/2 oz Edam cheese, grated
1 tablespoon chopped fresh parsley
freshly ground black pepper
1 teaspoon dried oregano

SERVES 4
Per serving: **Energy** 185 kcal/775 kJ
Fat 4 g
Fibre 8 g

Cook the cannelloni tubes in boiling water for 5 minutes.

Meanwhile drain one can of tomatoes and chop them. Mix with the breadcrumbs, cheese, parsley and pepper to taste.

Drain the cannelloni tubes and dry on absorbent kitchen paper. Fill with the cheese mixture and arrange in a lightly oiled ovenproof dish. Chop the tomatoes from the second can with their juice and pour over the cannelloni. Sprinkle the oregano on top.

Cook in a preheated moderate oven (180°C, 350°F, Gas Mark 4) for 30 minutes.

TOMATO AND WALNUT PASTA CASSEROLE

100 g/4 oz short-cut wholemeal macaroni
1 × 400 g (14 oz) can tomatoes
1 tablespoon grated onion
2 bay leaves
freshly ground black pepper
75 g/3 oz Edam cheese, grated
100 g/4 oz walnuts, chopped

SERVES 4
Per serving: **Energy** 280 kcal/1185 kJ
Fat 17 g
Fibre 5 g

Cook the macaroni in boiling water until tender.

Meanwhile place the tomatoes with their juice, the onion, bay leaves and pepper to taste in a saucepan. Bring to the boil, mashing the tomatoes with a spoon to break them up, and simmer until the mixture is thick.

Drain the macaroni thoroughly. Discard the bay leaves from the tomato sauce.

Make alternate layers of macaroni, tomato sauce, cheese and walnuts in a lightly oiled ovenproof dish, ending with tomato sauce and cheese. Cook in a preheated moderately hot oven (200°C, 400°F, Gas Mark 6) for about 25 minutes or until bubbling and the top is golden brown. Serve hot.

BROAD BEAN AND EGG CASSEROLE

450 g/1 lb frozen broad beans
3 hard-boiled eggs, sliced
40 g/1½ oz margarine
40 g/1½ oz plain wholemeal flour
450 ml/¾ pint skimmed milk
freshly ground black pepper

40 g/1½ oz Edam cheese, grated
5 tablespoons fresh wholemeal breadcrumbs

SERVES 4
Per serving: **Energy** 270 kcal/1125 kJ
Fat 15 g
Fibre 3 g

Cook the beans according to the directions on the packet. Drain well.

Place half the beans in an ovenproof dish and cover with the egg slices. Top with the remaining beans.

Melt the margarine in a saucepan. Stir in the flour and cook for 2 minutes, then gradually stir in the milk. Bring to the boil,

stirring, and simmer until thickened. Season to taste with pepper.

Pour the sauce over the beans. Mix together the cheese and breadcrumbs and scatter over the top. Cook in a preheated hot oven (220°C, 425°F, Gas Mark 7) for 15 minutes or until the top is golden brown. Serve hot.

CRUNCHY BAKED BEAN AND TOMATO CASSEROLE

225 g/8 oz white haricot beans, soaked overnight in cold water
225 g/8 oz tomatoes, sliced
1 medium onion, grated
2 teaspoons tomato purée
1 garlic clove, crushed
4 tablespoons chicken stock
2 tablespoons dry cider

freshly ground black pepper
TOPPING
100 g/4 oz wholemeal breadcrumbs

SERVES 4
Per serving: **Energy** 220 kcal/925 kJ
     Fat 2 g
     Fibre 18 g

Drain the beans and put in a saucepan with sufficient water to cover them by 2.5 cm/1 inch. Bring to the boil and boil rapidly for 10 minutes. Cover and simmer for about 1 hour or until tender. Drain.

Arrange the beans and tomatoes in layers in a 900 ml (2 pint) ovenproof dish. Mix

the remaining ingredients together and pour over the beans. Cook in a preheated moderate oven (160°C, 325°F, Gas Mark 3) for 45 minutes. Then sprinkle the breadcrumbs thickly over the top and place the dish under a preheated moderately hot grill to bubble and brown.

SPINACH AND MUSHROOM BAKE

1 × 225 g (8 oz) packet frozen chopped spinach, thawed and well drained
1 tablespoon lemon juice
freshly ground black pepper
4 rashers lean bacon, rinded, grilled and chopped
2 tablespoons olive oil
175 g/6 oz mushrooms, sliced
2 eggs

2 tablespoons plain unsweetened yogurt, stabilized (page 8)
75 g/3 oz Edam cheese, grated

SERVES 4
Per serving: **Energy** 225 kcal/940 kJ
     Fat 17 g
     Fibre 5 g

Mix the spinach with the lemon juice and pepper to taste. Fold in the bacon. Spread the mixture over the bottom of an ovenproof dish.

Heat the oil in a frying pan. Add the mushrooms and cook until tender. Arrange the mushrooms over the spinach mixture.

Beat the eggs lightly with the yogurt and

pepper to taste. Stir in the cheese. Pour over the mushrooms.

Cook in a preheated moderately hot oven (200°C, 400°F, Gas Mark 6) for 25 minutes. Serve hot.

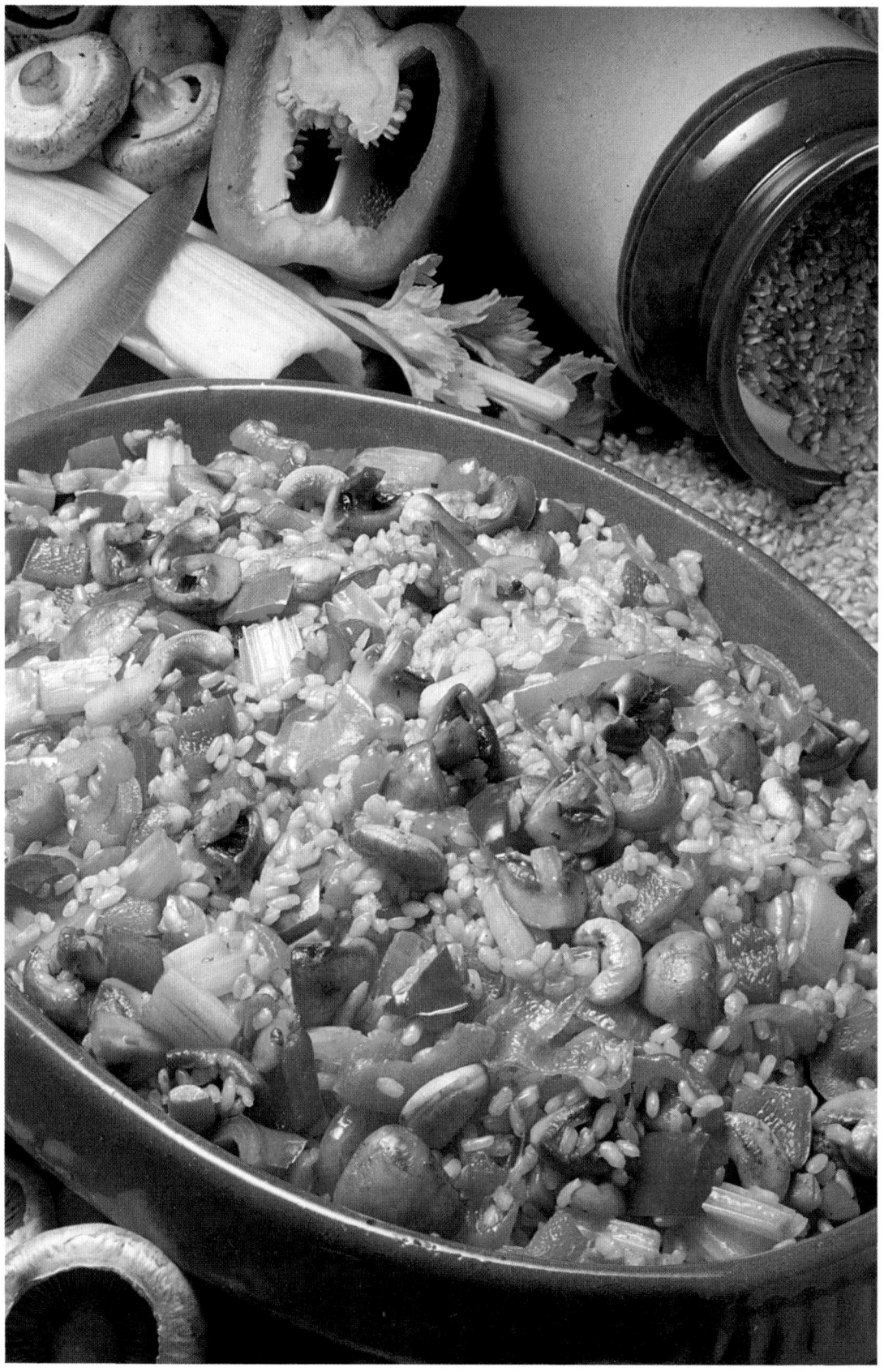

MUSHROOM AND NUT PILAFF

3 tablespoons olive oil
225 g/8 oz long-grain brown rice
1 medium onion, sliced
1 garlic clove, crushed
2 celery sticks, chopped
1 red pepper, cored, seeded and chopped
1 green pepper, cored, seeded and chopped
100 g/4 oz cashew nuts, chopped

175 g/6 oz button mushrooms, quartered
freshly ground black pepper

SERVES 4
Per serving: **Energy** 415 kcal/1735 kJ
            Fat 22 g
            Fibre 6 g

Heat 1 tablespoon of the oil in a large pan and cook the rice for 2–3 minutes. Cover with boiling water and cook for 45 minutes, then drain well.

Heat the remaining oil in a large pan and cook the onion until transparent. Add the garlic, celery, peppers, nuts and mushrooms and cook together for 5–7 minutes. Add the cooked rice and seasoning and simmer gently, stirring occasionally, until heated through.

Serve the pilaff with a green salad.

WHOLEMEAL PIZZA

15 g/½ oz fresh yeast or 1½ teaspoons dried
    yeast and ½ teaspoon caster sugar
6–7 tablespoons warm skimmed milk
225 g/8 oz plain wholemeal flour
freshly ground black pepper
25 g/1 oz margarine
TOPPING
1 medium onion, chopped
2 teaspoons olive oil
50 g/2 oz lean bacon, grilled and chopped
450 g/1 lb spinach

pinch of grated nutmeg
½ teaspoon lemon juice
225 g/8 oz tomatoes, sliced
50 g/2 oz black olives, halved
75 g/3 oz Mozzarella cheese, sliced
¼ teaspoon dried oregano

SERVES 6
Per serving: **Energy** 235 kcal/980 kJ
            Fat 7 g
            Fibre 9 g

Dissolve the fresh yeast in the warm milk, or dissolve the sugar in the warm milk and sprinkle the dried yeast on top. Leave the yeast in a warm place for 10 minutes or until frothy.

Mix together the flour and a little pepper and then rub in the margarine. Make a well in the centre and pour in the yeast mixture. Stir well until the mixture forms a ball. Knead on a lightly floured surface for 5 minutes. Place dough in an oiled polythene bag and leave in a warm place for 1 hour until doubled in size.

Meanwhile cook the onion in the oil until tender and add the cooked bacon. Remove from the heat and cool.

Wash the spinach thoroughly and remove the stalks. Cook the spinach for 2 minutes in boiling water seasoned with the nutmeg and lemon juice. Drain thoroughly and cool.

Turn the dough on to a lightly floured board and knead again for 1 minute. Roll out to a 28cm/11 inch round and place on a baking sheet lined with non-stick silicone paper. Cover the base with the spinach, add the bacon and onion. Top with the sliced tomatoes, olives and cheese and sprinkle over the oregano.

Cook the pizza in a preheated moderately hot oven (200°C, 400°F, Gas Mark 6) for 25 minutes.

OPPOSITE: MUSHROOM AND NUT PILAFF

NOODLES WITH ANCHOVY SAUCE

1 tablespoon oil
1 medium onion, chopped
1 garlic clove, crushed
1 × 50 g (2 oz) can anchovy fillets, drained,
    wiped and chopped
2 tablespoons chopped fresh parsley
1 tablespoon chopped fresh fennel
1 × 400 g (14 oz) can tomatoes

3 tablespoons sultanas
freshly ground black pepper
450 g / 1 lb wholemeal noodles

SERVES 6

Per serving:	Energy	315 kcal / 1320 kJ
	Fat	5 g
	Fibre	9 g

Heat the oil in a saucepan. Add the onion and garlic and fry until softened. Stir in the anchovies, parsley, fennel, tomatoes with their juice, sultanas and pepper to taste. Simmer for 20 minutes, stirring the sauce-pan gently occasionally.

Meanwhile, cook the noodles in boiling water until just tender. Drain well and return to the pan. Add the anchovy sauce and toss together. Serve hot.

COURGETTES WITH CORN

8 courgettes
1 tablespoon olive oil
1 medium onion, chopped
1 × 200 g (7 oz) can sweetcorn, drained
100 g / 4 oz Edam cheese, grated
50 g / 2 oz walnuts, chopped
freshly ground black pepper

SERVES 6

Per serving:	Energy	165 kcal / 700 kJ
	Fat	11 g
	Fibre	7 g

Cut the courgettes in half lengthways, scoop out the flesh and chop finely. Blanch the shells in boiling water for 2 minutes and drain well.

Heat the oil in a pan and fry the onion and courgette flesh for 5 minutes, until softened, then add the remaining ingredients and mix well.

Arrange the courgette shells in a shallow ovenproof casserole, fill with the mixture, cover and bake in a preheated oven, (190°C, 375°F, Gas Mark 5) for 40 minutes.

FRUIT SANDWICH

2 slices wholemeal bread
1 tablespoon Date spread (page 121)
1 small orange, peeled and segmented
1 teaspoon chopped walnuts

MAKES 1

Per sandwich:	Energy	255 kcal / 1070 kJ
	Fat	7 g
	Fibre	9 g

Spread both slices of bread with the Date spread and fill the sandwich with the orange segments and the walnuts.

VARIATION
Spread the slices of bread with Crunchy peanut butter (page 120). Cover one slice with 1 small banana, peeled and thinly sliced. Sprinkle 2 teaspoons of raisins over the banana.

Per sandwich:	Energy	330 kcal / 1380 kJ
	Fat	7 g
	Fibre	9 g

TOASTED TURKEY SANDWICHES

225 g/8 oz cooked turkey meat, diced
2 tablespoons plain unsweetened yogurt,
  stabilized (page 8)
1 celery stick, finely chopped
75 g/3 oz Edam cheese, grated
1 tablespoon diced red pepper
1 × 200 g (7 oz) can sweetcorn kernels, drained

8 slices wholemeal bread
25 g/1 oz melted margarine

SERVES 4
Per serving: **Energy** 335 kcal/1485 kJ
　　　　　　 Fat 13 g
　　　　　　 Fibre 8 g

Mix together the turkey, yogurt, celery, cheese, red pepper and corn. Use to make four sandwiches with the wholemeal bread. Arrange on the grill pan and brush the tops with melted margarine. Grill until the bread is browned, then turn over and brush the sandwich bottoms with more melted margarine. Continue grilling until the other sides of the sandwiches are browned. Serve hot.

VARIATION
Cooked chicken meat may be substituted for the turkey.

QUICK SARDINE PIZZAS

2 wholemeal muffins, split in half
tomato purée
1 × 100 g (4 oz) can sardines, drained and
  wiped
freshly ground black pepper
4 processed cheese slices
dried oregano
8 black olives, stoned

SERVES 4
Per serving: **Energy** 160 kcal/670 kJ
　　　　　　 Fat 7 g
　　　　　　 Fibre 3 g

Spread the cut surfaces of the muffins with the tomato purée. Top with the sardines and sprinkle with pepper. Lay a slice of cheese on top of each 'pizza' and sprinkle with oregano. Garnish with the olives.

Arrange the pizzas on a baking sheet lined with non-stick silicone paper. Cook in a preheated moderately hot oven (200°C, 400°F, Gas Mark 6) for 15 minutes. Alternatively, the pizzas may be cooked under the grill, which would take about 10 minutes. Serve hot.

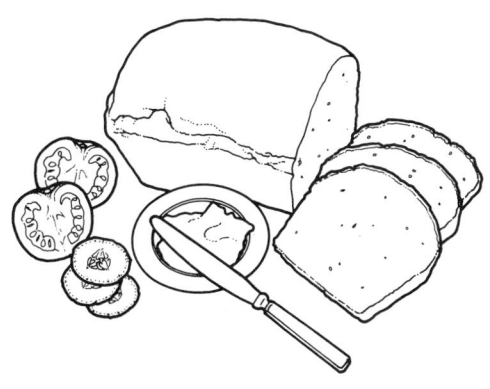

Baking

WHOLEMEAL BREAD

1.5 kg/3 lb 100% stoneground wholemeal flour
25 g/1 oz bran
25 g/1 oz margarine
25 g/1 oz fresh yeast
1 teaspoon muscovado sugar
900 ml/1½ pints warm water
2 tablespoons malt extract

TOPPING
skimmed milk
2 tablespoons cracked wheat

MAKES 4 loaves
Per loaf: Energy 1295 kcal/5435 kJ
       Fat 13 g
       Fibre 39 g

Mix the flour and bran together in a bowl and rub in the fat. Blend the yeast with the sugar and 3 tablespoons of the water. Add the yeast liquid to the dry ingredients with the remaining water and the malt extract. Draw the ingredients together and beat until the mixture comes cleanly away from the sides of the bowl.

Turn out on to a floured surface and knead the dough for 8 minutes until it is smooth and elastic. Place in a lightly oiled bowl, cover with a damp cloth and leave in a warm place to rise until doubled in size.

Turn out on to a floured surface and knead again for 2 minutes, then cut into 4 pieces. Shape into loaves and place each loaf in a lightly oiled 450 g (1 lb) loaf tin. Cover and leave in a warm place to prove until the dough rises to the top of the tins.

Brush with milk and sprinkle with cracked wheat. Bake in a preheated hot oven (230°C, 450°F, Gas Mark 8) for 10 minutes, then reduce the heat to 190°C, 375°F, Gas Mark 5 for 30 minutes, or until the bread sounds hollow when tapped underneath. Cool on a wire tray.

FIG LOAF

100 g/4 oz All-Bran
75 g/3 oz muscovado sugar
100 g/4 oz dried figs, chopped
2 teaspoons black treacle
300 ml/½ pint skimmed milk
100 g/4 oz self-raising wholemeal flour

MAKES 1 loaf
Per loaf: Energy 1230 kcal/5175 kJ
       Fat 8 g
       Fibre 55 g

Put the All-Bran, sugar, figs, black treacle and skimmed milk into a bowl. Mix well together and leave to stand for 30 minutes. Sift in the flour, mixing well. Put the mixture into a 450 g (1 lb) loaf tin lined with non-stick silicone paper. Bake in a preheated moderate oven (180°C, 350°F, Gas Mark 4) for 45–60 minutes. Turn out of the tin and allow to cool on a wire tray.

OPPOSITE: FIG LOAF

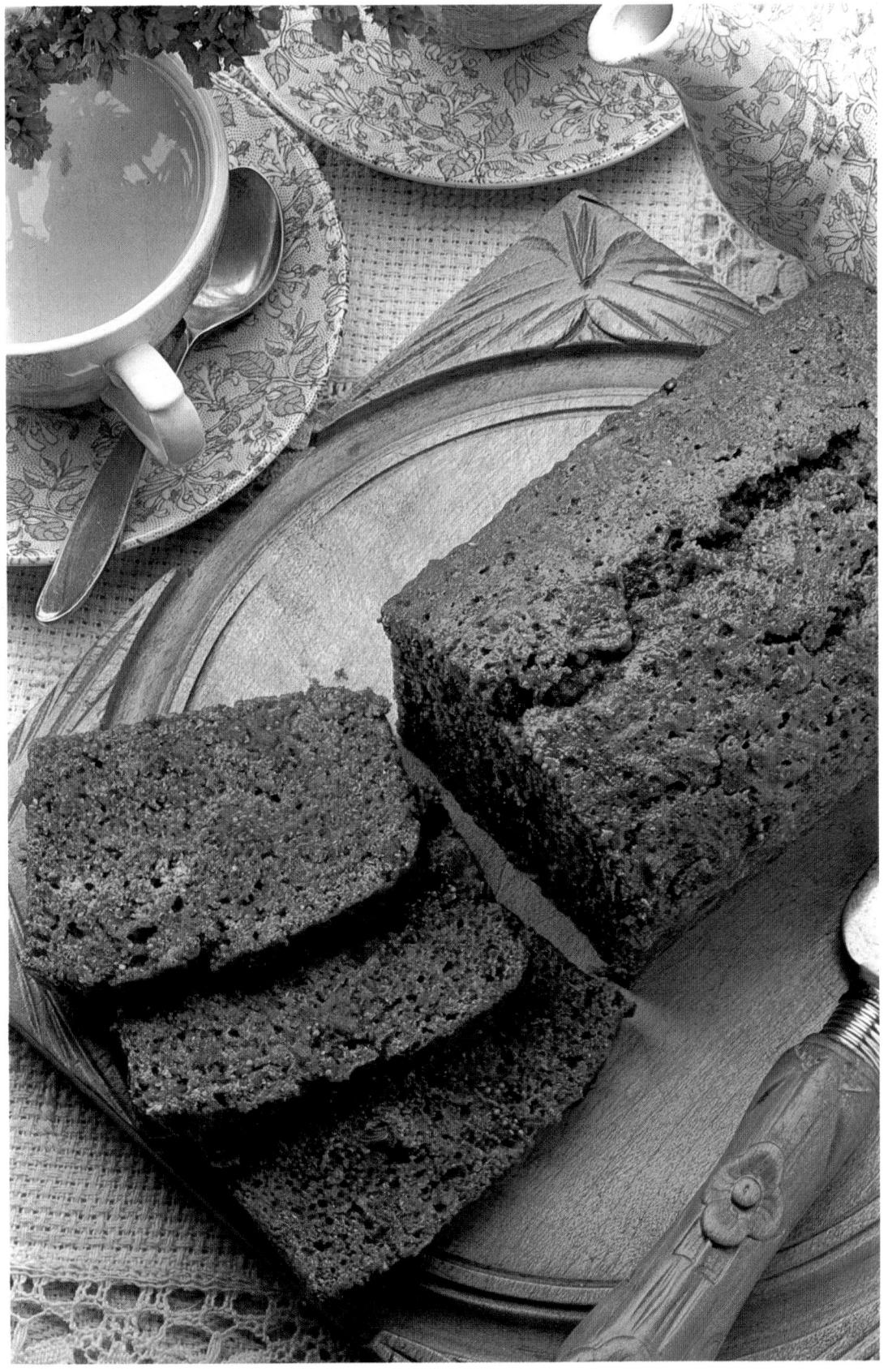

FRUIT BRAN LOAF

150 g / 5 oz bran cereal
275 g / 10 oz mixed sultanas and seedless raisins
300 ml / ½ pint skimmed milk or buttermilk
150 g / 5 oz plain wholemeal flour
1 tablespoon baking powder
pinch of ground mixed spice
grated rind of ½ orange (optional)
1 egg, beaten

MAKES 1 loaf
Per loaf: Energy 1750 kcal / 7340 kJ
Fat 17 g
Fibre 74 g

Put the bran cereal, dried fruit and milk or buttermilk in a large mixing bowl, cover with a plate and leave to soak overnight.

The next day, sift the flour, baking powder and spice into the bowl, then tip in any bran left in the sieve. Add the orange rind, if used. Make a well in the centre, add the egg and mix thoroughly.

Put the mixture into a 1 kg (2 lb) loaf tin lined with non-stick silicone paper. Bake in a preheated moderate oven (180°C, 350°F, Gas Mark 4) for 1 hour or until a skewer inserted into the centre of the loaf comes out clean. Loosen the loaf with a palette knife and turn out of the tin on to a wire tray to cool.

COFFEE CHESTNUT BREAD

225 g / 8 oz self-raising wholemeal flour
½ teaspoon baking powder
2 tablespoons instant coffee powder
50 g / 2 oz margarine
40 g / 1½ oz caster sugar
100 g / 4 oz canned unsweetened whole
*   chestnuts, drained and chopped*
50 g / 2 oz dates, stoned and chopped

1 egg, beaten
150 ml / ¼ pint skimmed milk

MAKES 1 loaf
Per loaf: Energy 1675 kcal / 7045 kJ
Fat 53 g
Fibre 33 g

Sift the flour, baking powder and coffee into a bowl, tipping in any bran left in the sieve. Rub in the margarine and stir in the sugar. Mix in the chestnuts and dates. Make a well in the centre and add the egg and milk. Combine all the ingredients

thoroughly. Place in a greased 450 g (1 lb) loaf tin.

Cook in a preheated moderate oven (180°C, 350°F, Gas Mark 4) for 45 minutes. Leave to cool in the tin for 10 minutes, then turn out on to a wire tray to finish cooling.

BANANA AND NUT TEA BREAD

200 g / 7 oz plain wholemeal flour
1 teaspoon baking powder
50 g / 2 oz margarine
50 g / 2 oz muscovado sugar
1 egg
4 tablespoons skimmed milk

2 large ripe bananas, sliced
25 g / 1 oz walnuts, chopped

MAKES 1 loaf
Per loaf: Energy 1530 kcal / 6425 kJ
Fat 65 g
Fibre 25 g

Line a 450 g (1 lb) loaf tin with non-stick silicone paper.

Sift the flour and baking powder into a large bowl. Rub in the margarine and add the sugar. Whip the egg, milk and bananas together and mix thoroughly with the dry ingredients. Add the nuts. Turn into the prepared loaf tin. Bake in a preheated moderate oven (180°C, 350°F, Gas Mark 4) for about 1 hour. Cool for 5 minutes in the loaf tin before turning on to a wire tray to cool completely.

COFFEE, APPLE AND DATE LOAF

350 g/12 oz plain wholemeal flour
1 tablespoon baking powder
50 g/2 oz caster sugar
1 tablespoon instant coffee powder
1 egg, beaten
300 ml/½ pint skimmed milk
2 dessert apples, cored and chopped
100 g/4 oz dates, stoned and chopped

MAKES 1 loaf
Per loaf: Energy 1830 kcal/7680 kJ
          Fat 13 g
          Fibre 45 g

Combine the flour, baking powder, sugar and coffee. Beat together the egg and milk and add to the flour mixture with the apples and dates. Mix well. Pour into a 450 g (1 lb) loaf tin lined with non-stick silicone paper.

Cook in a preheated moderate oven (180°C, 350°F, Gas Mark 4) for 1 hour or until a knife inserted in the centre comes out clean. Allow to cool in the tin.

AVOCADO BREAD

50 g/2 oz margarine
50 g/2 oz muscovado sugar
200 g/7 oz plain wholemeal flour
1 teaspoon baking powder
1 teaspoon bicarbonate of soda
½ teaspoon ground nutmeg
½ teaspoon ground cinnamon
2 eggs
100 ml/3½ fl oz buttermilk

1 × 225 g (8 oz) avocado, stoned and peeled
  (175 g/6 oz flesh)
25 g/1 oz Brazil nuts, chopped
1 teaspoon grated lemon rind

MAKES 1 loaf
Per loaf: Energy 1915 kcal/8035 kJ
          Fat 110 g
          Fibre 25 g

Line a 450 g (1 lb) loaf tin with non-stick silicone paper.

Cream the margarine and beat in the sugar. Sift the flour, baking powder, bicarbonate of soda and spices into a bowl. Whip the eggs, buttermilk and avocado flesh together. Add the flour and egg mixtures alternately to the creamed margarine and sugar, beating well between each addition. Stir the nuts and lemon rind into the mixture. Turn into the prepared loaf tin and bake in a preheated moderate oven (160°C, 325°F, Gas Mark 3) for about 1 hour. Cool in the tin for 5 minutes before turning on to a wire tray to cool completely. Serve this bread with salads.

COTTAGE CHEESE AND WALNUT TEA BREAD

200 g/7 oz cottage cheese, sieved
100 g/4 oz muscovado sugar
3 eggs, beaten
75 g/3 oz walnuts, chopped
50 g/2 oz chopped mixed peel (optional)
200 g/7 oz self-raising wholemeal flour
1 teaspoon baking powder

MAKES 1 loaf
Per loaf: Energy 1810 kcal/7610 kJ
Fat 65 g
Fibre 23 g

Line a 600 g (1½ lb) loaf tin with non-stick silicone paper. Cream together the cottage cheese and sugar and beat in the eggs. Stir in the walnuts and peel if used. Sift in the flour and baking powder and fold into the mixture. Turn into the prepared tin. Bake in a preheated moderate oven (180°C, 350°F, Gas Mark 4) for 1 hour until well risen and golden brown. Leave in the tin for 5 minutes, then turn out and cool on a wire tray.

Serve the tea bread sliced.

SULTANA AND NUT CRESCENTS, COMPLETED AND (FAR RIGHT) IN PREPARATION

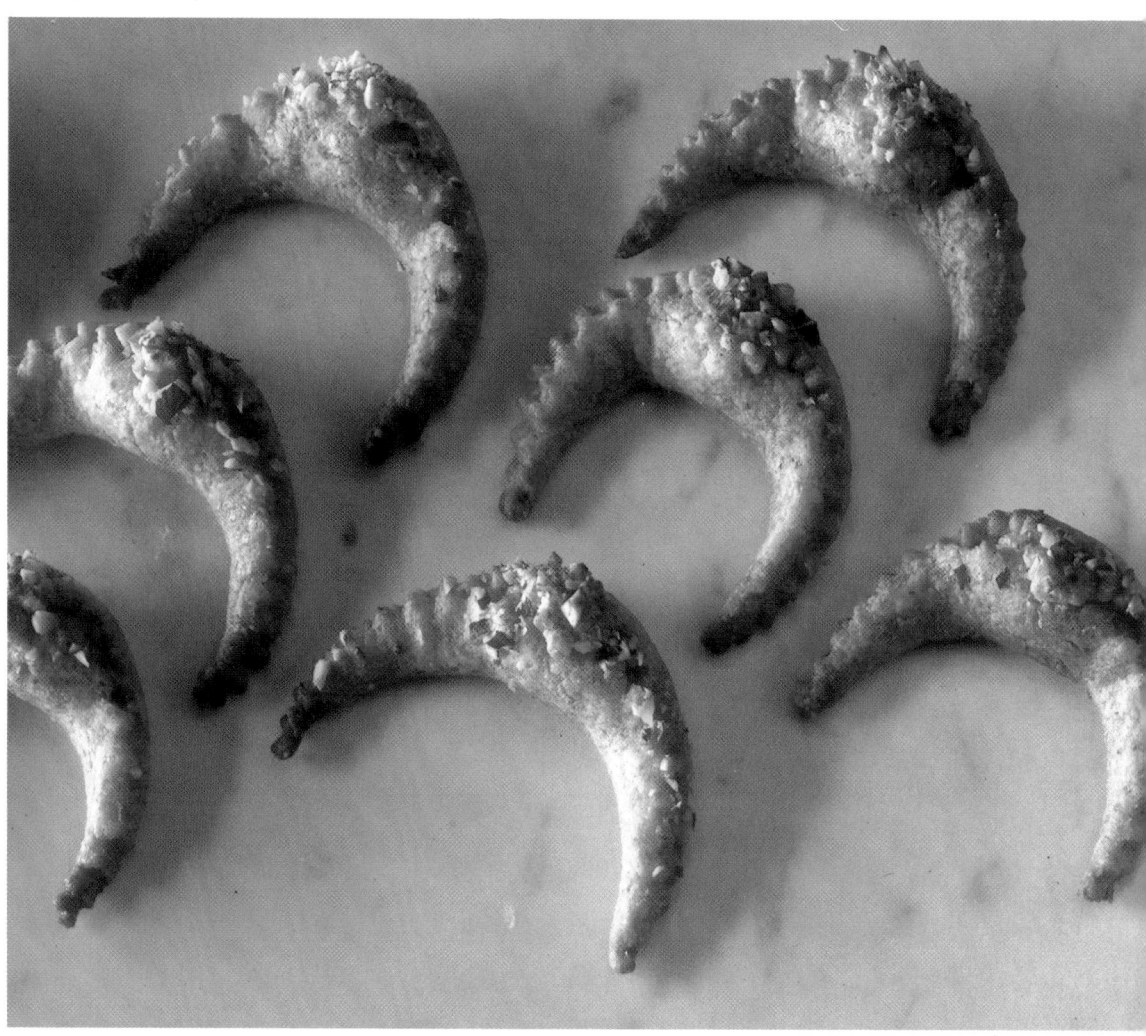

SULTANA AND NUT CRESCENTS

100 g / 4 oz plain wholemeal flour
100 g / 4 oz margarine
100 g / 4 oz quark or low-fat soft cheese
FILLING
40 g / 1½ oz sultanas
2 teaspoons caster sugar
25 g / 1 oz hazelnuts, chopped
¼ teaspoon ground cinnamon (optional)

TO FINISH
100 ml / 3½ fl oz skimmed milk
25 g / 1 oz hazelnuts, finely chopped

MAKES about 24 crescents
Per crescent: Energy 55 kcal / 240 kJ
    Fat 4 g
    Fibre 1 g

Sift the flour into a bowl and rub in the margarine. Add the cheese and mix to a dough. Chill.

Roll out the dough and cut into triangles. Mix together the filling ingredients and put a small spoonful of filling in the centre of each triangle. Roll them up from the wide side. Brush each crescent with a little milk to seal the edges; sprinkle with nuts and cinnamon. Arrange on a baking sheet lined with non-stick silicone paper, curving slightly into crescents.

Bake in a preheated moderately hot oven (200°C, 390°F, Gas Mark 5) for 15 minutes.

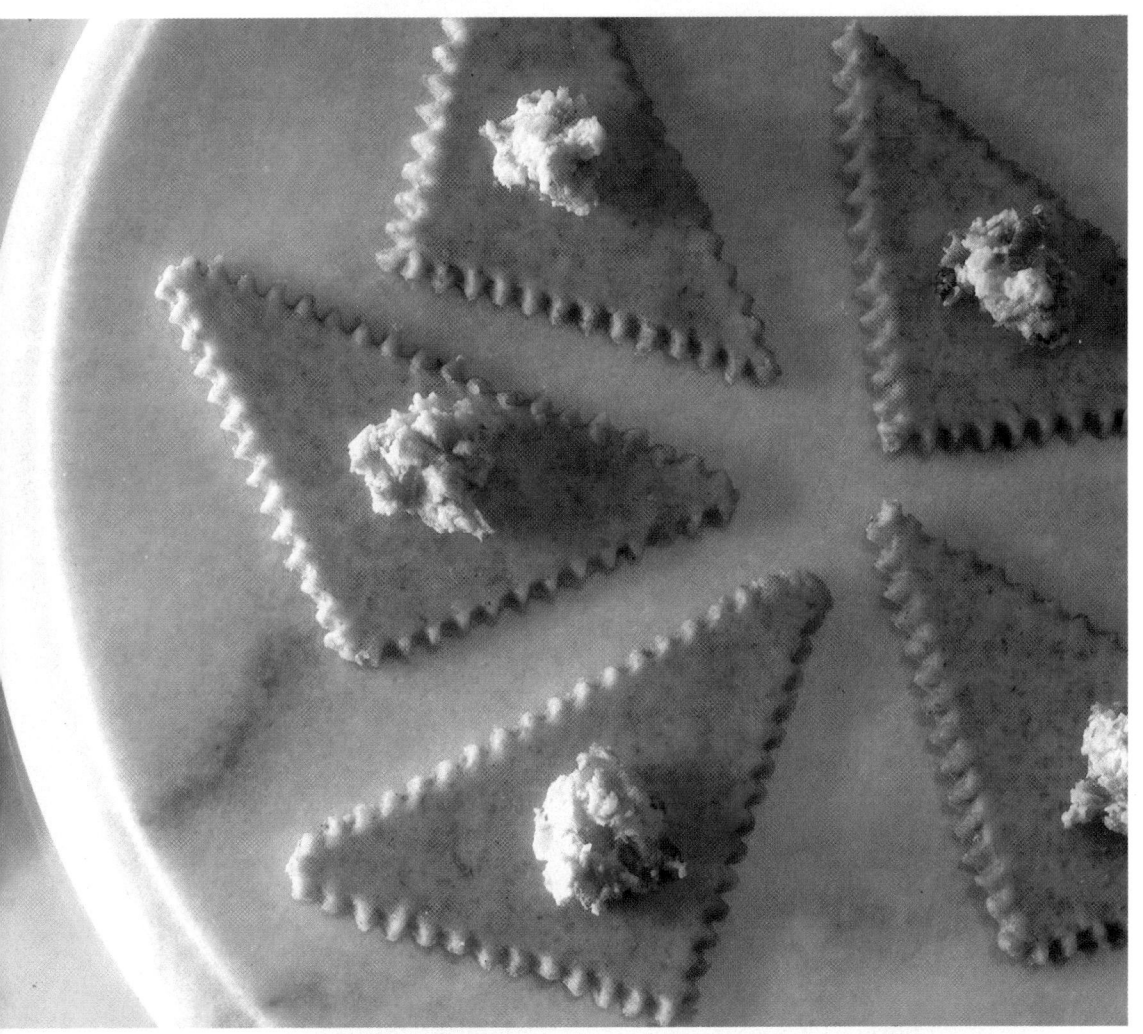

PEANUT BUTTER BISCUITS

75 g/3 oz Crunchy peanut butter (page 120)
25 g/1 oz margarine
grated rind of ½ orange
40 g/1½ oz caster sugar
40 g/1½ oz light soft brown sugar
½ beaten egg
40 g/1½ oz raisins or sultanas, chopped
100 g/4 oz self-raising wholemeal flour

MAKES 16–20 biscuits
Per biscuit: Energy 80 kcal/330 kJ
           Fat   4 g
           Fibre 1 g

Put the peanut butter, margarine, orange rind and sugars into a bowl and beat until light and fluffy. Beat in the egg, then add the dried fruit and flour and mix to a fairly firm dough. Roll into balls about the size of a walnut and place well apart on ungreased baking sheets. Slightly flatten each one using a fork or blunt knife and mark with a criss-cross pattern.

Bake in a preheated moderate oven (180°C, 350°F, Gas Mark 4) for about 25 minutes or until well risen and golden brown. Remove to a wire tray to cool. Store in an airtight container.

CHEESE AND ALMOND BISCUITS

75 g/3 oz plain wholemeal flour
½ teaspoon paprika
freshly ground black pepper
40 g/1½ oz margarine
40 g/1½ oz ground almonds
40 g/1½ oz grated Parmesan cheese
1 egg yolk

MAKES about 24 biscuits
Per biscuit: Energy 40 kcal/170 kJ
           Fat   3 g
           Fibre 1 g

Sift the flour, paprika and pepper into a mixing bowl. Cut the margarine into the flour and rub in to a breadcrumb consistency. Mix in the ground almonds and grated cheese. Stir in the egg yolk and mix into a soft dough, adding a little water if necessary.

Roll out to 5 mm/¼ inch thick. Cut out 5 cm/2 inch rounds and place on a baking sheet lined with non-stick silicone paper. Bake in a preheated moderate oven (180°C, 350°F, Gas Mark 4) for 10 minutes or until set and golden brown. Remove from the oven and cool slightly before lifting from the baking sheet. Serve warm or cold.

HAZELNUT OATMEAL BISCUITS

225 g/8 oz wholemeal flour
75 g/3 oz medium oatmeal
75 g/3 oz bran
75 g/3 oz ground hazelnuts
50 g/2 oz muscovado sugar
100 g/4 oz margarine
about 150 ml/¼ pint water

MAKES about 48 biscuits
Per biscuit: Energy 50 kcal/215 kJ
           Fat   3 g
           Fibre 1 g

Mix together the flour, oatmeal, bran, ground hazelnuts and sugar and rub in the margarine. Mix in enough water to make a stiff dough.

Roll out the dough to 1 cm/½ inch thick and cut out 6 cm/2½ inch rounds. Place them on baking sheets lined with non-stick silicone paper. Bake in a preheated moderate oven (180°C, 350°F, Gas Mark 4) for 25 minutes. Cool on a wire tray.

DATE AND APPLE CRUNCHIES

100 g/4 oz margarine
75 g/3 oz muscovado sugar
2 tablespoons golden syrup
2 teaspoons grated lemon rind
175 g/6 oz rolled oats
50 g/2 oz wholemeal flour
1 teaspoon baking powder
100 g/4 oz stoned dates, chopped

1 tablespoon lemon juice
225 g/8 oz dessert apples, cored and finely
*   chopped or coarsely grated*

MAKES 16 crunchies
Per crunchy: Energy 145 kcal/605 kJ
**   Fat** 6 g
**   Fibre** 2 g

Melt the fat with the sugar, golden syrup and grated lemon rind in a saucepan over a gentle heat. Stir well and do not allow to boil. Set aside to cool. Mix together the rolled oats, flour and baking powder. Stir in the cooled liquid ingredients and mix very thoroughly.

Turn half the mixture into an 18 cm (7 inch) square tin lined with non-stick silicone paper. Spread out evenly and press down with a wooden spoon. Mix the chopped dates and apples with the lemon juice and spread over the oat mixture. Cover with the remaining mixture and press down firmly.

Bake in a preheated moderate oven (180°C, 35°F, Gas Mark 4) for 20–30 minutes until firm and golden. Remove from the oven and cut into 16 equal portions.

Allow to cool, then remove from the tin and cool on a wire tray. When cold store in an airtight container.

HERB BISCUITS

50 g/2 oz plain wholemeal flour
25 g/1 oz margarine
pinch of cayenne
50 g/2 oz Edam cheese, grated
½ teaspoon caraway seeds or dried dill seed
½ teaspoon Dijon mustard
1 egg yolk
1 tablespoon iced water

MAKES about 20 biscuits
Per biscuit: Energy 25 kcal/115 kJ
**   Fat** 2 g
**   Fibre** negligible

Sift the flour into a bowl and rub in the margarine in small pieces. Add the cayenne and mix in the grated cheese with the blade of a knife. (Alternatively, all this can be done in a mixer or food processor.) Stir in the caraway seeds (or dill). Stir the mustard into the lightly beaten egg yolk and stir into the mixture. Add enough of the iced water to give a soft but firm dough.

Wrap loosely in cling film and chill for 1 hour. Roll out on a floured board until about 3 mm/⅛ inch thick and cut into small rounds. Lay the biscuits on a baking sheet lined with non-stick silicone paper and bake for 7 minutes in a moderately hot oven (200°C, 400°F, Gas Mark 6) or until golden brown and puffed up. Serve immediately, with a thick soup.

ONION BISCUITS

225 g/8 oz plain wholemeal flour
freshly ground black pepper
100 g/4 oz margarine
1 medium onion, finely grated
1 egg, beaten
beaten egg to glaze
poppy seeds (optional)

MAKES about 24 biscuits
Per biscuit: Energy 64 kcal/275 kJ
Fat 4 g
Fibre 1 g

Sift the flour and pepper into a bowl and rub in the margarine. Add the onion and egg and mix to a stiff dough, adding a little cold water if necessary. Roll out the dough and cut into 5 cm/2 inch squares. Place on baking sheets lined with non-stick silicone paper and brush with beaten egg. Sprinkle with poppy seeds, if liked.

Bake in a preheated moderately hot oven (200°C, 400°F, Gas Mark 6) for 15–20 minutes.

Serve the biscuits warm or cold.

CARROT BUNS

200 g/7 oz plain wholemeal flour
2 teaspoons baking powder
6 tablespoons plain unsweetened yogurt
1 tablespoon molasses
2 eggs
50 g/2 oz grated carrots

MAKES 12 buns
Per bun: Energy 75 kcal/305 kJ
Fat 1 g
Fibre 2 g

Sift flour and baking powder into a large bowl. Whip the remaining ingredients together and combine with the flour. Divide the mixture evenly into 6 cm/2½ inch diameter non-stick bun tins. Bake in a preheated moderately hot oven (190°C, 375°F, Gas Mark 5) for 15–20 minutes. Serve the buns hot.

Split and fill them with Date spread (page 121), if liked.

OATMEAL BUNS

100 g/4 oz self-raising wholemeal flour, sifted
100 g/4 oz rolled oats
50 g/2 oz margarine
1 tablespoon clear honey
120 ml/4 fl oz strong black coffee
120 ml/4 fl oz skimmed milk
100 g/4 oz blanched almonds, chopped

MAKES 12 buns
Per bun: Energy 145 kcal/605 kJ
Fat 9 g
Fibre 3 g

Combine the flour and oats in a bowl. Melt the margarine with the honey and coffee in a small saucepan and stir in the milk. Heat until almost boiling, but do not allow to boil. Add to the dry ingredients with the almonds and mix well. Place the mixture in lightly oiled patty tins.

Cook in a preheated moderately hot oven (200°C, 400°F, Gas Mark 6) for 30 minutes. Leave for 5 minutes, then turn out on to a wire tray.

Serve the buns warm or cold.

SCONES

225 g/8 oz self-raising wholemeal flour
1½ teaspoons baking powder
25 g/1 oz margarine
1 tablespoon caster sugar
150 ml/¼ pint plain unsweetened yogurt

MAKES 16–18 scones
Per scone: Energy 60 kcal/260 kJ
Fat 2 g
Fibre 1 g

Sift the flour and baking powder into a bowl. Rub in the margarine, then stir in the sugar. Bind to a soft but not sticky dough with the yogurt.

Roll out the dough on a floured surface to about 4 cm/1½ inches thick and cut into 5 cm/2 inch rounds. Place these on a baking sheet lined with non-stick silicone paper.

Bake in a preheated very hot oven (230°C, 450°F, Gas Mark 8) for 8–10 minutes or until well risen and golden. Cool on a wire tray and serve warm.

VARIATIONS
SPICED TREACLE SCONES Follow the recipe for basic scones, sifting ¾ teaspoon ground mixed spice with the flour and replacing the sugar with 1 tablespoon black treacle added with the yogurt.

Per scone: Energy 60 kcal/260 kJ
Fat 2 g
Fibre 1 g

HONEY AND WALNUT SCONES Follow the recipe for basic scones, but omit the baking powder. Stir in 25 g/1 oz chopped walnuts with the sugar. Add to the dry ingredients 2–3 tablespoons only of yogurt, 1 beaten egg and 1 tablespoon thin honey.

Per scone: Energy 70 kcal/300 kJ
Fat 3 g
Fibre 1 g

DATE SCONES Follow the recipe for basic scones, but omit the baking powder and add 1 beaten egg with the yogurt. Work in 175 g/6 oz chopped stoned dates.

Per scone: Energy 90 kcal/380 kJ
Fat 2 g
Fibre 2 g

SWISS HAZELNUT AND CARROT CAKE

3 eggs, separated
100 g/4 oz caster sugar
120 g/4½ oz peeled carrots, grated
120 g/4½ oz hazelnuts, very finely chopped
2 teaspoons finely grated lemon rind
50 g/2 oz plain wholemeal flour
½ teaspoon baking powder

SERVES 6
Per serving: Energy 320 kcal/1340 kJ
Fat 16 g
Fibre 4 g

Line an 18 cm (7 inch) square tin with non-stick silicone paper.

Whisk the egg yolks and the sugar until thick and creamy. Stir in the carrots, hazelnuts and lemon rind. Sift the flour and baking powder and fold in. Whisk the egg whites until they form stiff peaks, then carefully fold into the mixture. Turn into the cake tin and bake in a preheated oven (180°C, 350°F, Gas Mark 4) for 40–45 minutes. Leave in the tin for 2–3 minutes, then turn out on to a wire tray to cool.

CARROT AND ALMOND CAKE

5 eggs, separated
175 g/6 oz demerara sugar
grated rind of ½ orange
275 g/10 oz carrots, scrubbed and grated
275 g/10 oz ground almonds
100 g/4 oz plain wholemeal flour
1 tablespoon brandy or orange liqueur (Grand
    Marnier) or orange juice
TO FINISH
1 tablespoon demerara sugar
1 teaspoon ground cinnamon
25 g/1 oz flaked almonds

SERVES 6
Per serving: **Energy**   460 kcal/1930 kJ
             Fat   32 g
             Fibre   10 g

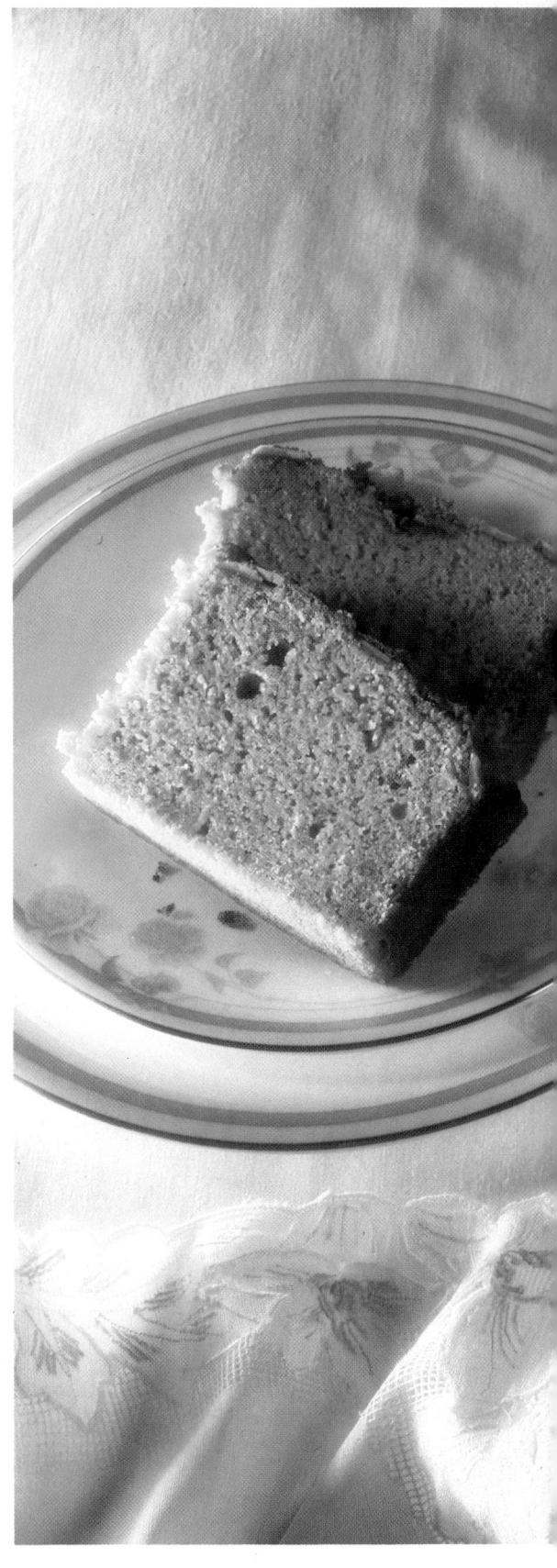

Beat the egg yolks with a wire whisk until frothy. Add the sugar gradually and beat until the mixture is pale and thick. Fold in the orange rind, carrots, almonds, flour and brandy, liqueur or orange juice. Beat the egg whites until stiff and fold into the cake mixture with a metal spoon. Pour the mixture into a 18 cm/7 inch square tin lined with non-stick silicone paper.

Mix together the demerara sugar and cinnamon and sprinkle over the surface. Scatter the flaked almonds on top. Bake in the centre of a preheated moderately hot oven (190°C, 375°F, Gas Mark 5) for 1 hour or until the cake is springy to the touch and a hot skewer inserted into the centre comes out clean.

Leave the cake to cool in the tin for about 15 minutes before turning it out on to a wire tray to cool. Store the cake in an airtight container in the refrigerator if intending to leave it for more than 3 days.

VARIATION

A more economical version of this cake can be made by reducing the ground almonds to 100 g/4 oz and increasing the flour to 275 g/10 oz, and the carrots to 350 g/12 oz. Add two drops of almond essence with the liqueur or orange juice and make the cake in the same way as described above.

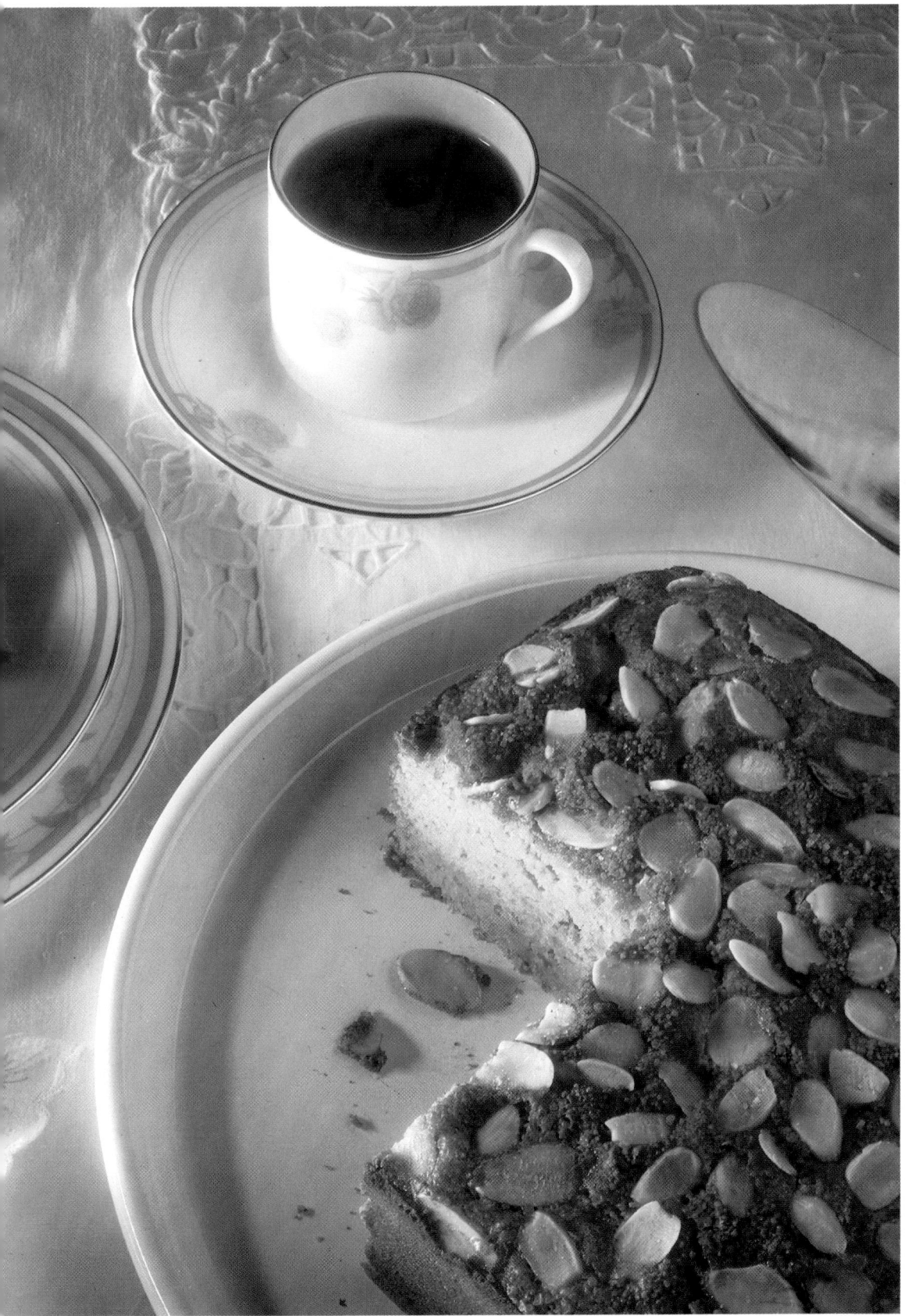

CARROT LOAF CAKE

225 g/8 oz wholemeal plain flour
pinch of ground allspice
1 teaspoon bicarbonate of soda
½ teaspoon cream of tartar
225 g/8 oz carrots, scrubbed and grated
100 g/4 oz unsalted peanuts, chopped
1 tablespoon golden syrup

2 eggs
175 ml/6 fl oz corn oil

SERVES 6
Per serving: **Energy** 515 kcal/2170 kJ
  Fat 40 g
  Fibre 6 g

Line a 1 kg (2 lb) loaf tin with non-stick silicone paper. Sift the flour, allspice, bicarbonate of soda and cream of tartar together into a mixing bowl. Stir in the carrots and 75 g/3 oz of the chopped peanuts.

Beat the golden syrup, eggs and oil together and stir them into the dry ingredients to make a soft dropping consistency. Spoon the mixture into the prepared tin, then sprinkle over the remaining peanuts.

Cook in a preheated moderate oven (180°C, 350°F, Gas Mark 4) for 1½ hours or until the loaf is well risen and shrinking away from the sides of the tin. Cool the loaf in the tin for 10 minutes, then turn out on to a wire tray to cool completely. Store for 24 hours before use: otherwise it may be difficult to cut.

APPLE AND POTATO CAKE

750 g/1½ lb floury potatoes, peeled
50 g/2 oz margarine
about 4 tablespoons self-raising wholemeal flour

3 dessert apples, peeled, cored and chopped
TO FINISH
1–2 tablespoons caster sugar

SERVES 4–6
4 servings
Per serving: **Energy** 355 kcal/1480 kJ
  Fat 11 g
  Fibre 7 g

6 servings
Per serving: **Energy** 235 kcal/990 kJ
  Fat 7 g
  Fibre 4 g

Boil the potatoes in water. Drain and cover with a clean cloth until dry and floury, but still very hot. Sieve through a mouli-légumes or wire sieve and weigh off 450 g/1 lb of potato.

Put the sieved potato in a warm mixing bowl and beat in the fat. Work in sufficient flour to make the dough manageable.

Divide the dough in half and pat or roll out into rounds of equal size just over 1 cm/½ inch thick. Place one round on a warmed non-stick griddle and spread with the chopped apple. Cover with the other round of dough and pinch the edges together all round.

Bake on the griddle over a moderate heat until brown underneath. Slide the lightly oiled base of a cake tin underneath, turn the cake over and cook the other side. Slide the cake on to a hot serving dish, fold back one half of the top and sprinkle the apples with sugar. Repeat with the other half of the cake and serve at once.

If no griddle is available, the cake can be cooked in a preheated moderately hot oven (200°C, 400°F, Gas Mark 6) for about 30 minutes without turning.

VARIATION
Use Bramley apples which become fluffy when cooked.

BANANA DROP SCONES

225 g / 8 oz plain wholemeal flour
1 teaspoon baking powder
1 egg
2 teaspoons muscovado sugar
2 small bananas
200 ml / 1/3 pint skimmed milk

MAKES about 18 scones
Per scone: **Energy** 55 kcal / 235 kJ
          Fat   1 g
          Fibre   2 g

Sift the flour and baking powder into a large bowl. Whip the remaining ingredients together until smoothly blended. Make a well in the centre of the flour mixture and pour in the liquid. Stir with a wooden spoon until the mixture forms a batter that drops easily from the lifted spoon. If necessary, add a little more skimmed milk.

Heat a non-stick pan over a moderate heat and drop spoonfuls of the batter on to it, using the back of the spoon to level the mixture to about 1 cm / 1/2 inch thickness. When bubbles cover the surface, turn over with a wooden spatula and cook the other side. Serve hot.

CORNMEAL MERINGUES

50 g / 2 oz cornmeal
350 ml / 12 fl oz cold water
4 egg whites

MAKES 12 meringues
Per meringue: **Energy** 17 kcal / 70 kJ
          Fat   negligible
          Fibre negligible

Combine the cornmeal with the water in a saucepan and boil for 3 minutes, stirring constantly. Whip the egg whites very stiffly and fold into the cornmeal mixture. Drop tablespoons of the mixture on to baking sheets lined with non-stick silicone paper. Bake in a preheated cool oven (140°C, 275°F, Gas Mark 1) for about 1½ hours or until the meringues have dried sufficiently to be lifted easily with a slice from the paper.

Serve the meringues warm with bean soups.

CORNMEAL WAFFLES

100 g / 4 oz plain wholemeal flour
100 g / 4 oz cornmeal
3 teaspoons baking powder
2 eggs, separated
300 ml / 1/2 pint skimmed milk
2 tablespoons olive oil

MAKES 8 waffles
Per waffle: **Energy** 145 kcal / 615 kJ
        Fat   6 g
        Fibre 1 g

Sift the flour, cornmeal and baking powder into a bowl. Combine the well-beaten egg yolks with the milk and add to the flour mixture, beating until smooth. Beat in the oil. Fold in stiffly beaten egg whites.

Pour some of the batter carefully into a preheated non-stick waffle iron. Leave over a moderate heat until the underside is brown, opening the waffle iron to check after 1–2 minutes. Turn the closed iron over and cook the other side.

COTTAGE CHEESE GRIDDLECAKES

25 g / 1 oz margarine, melted
100 g / 4 oz cottage cheese
2 eggs, beaten
50 g / 2 oz self-raising wholemeal flour
1 tablespoon skimmed milk

MAKES 10–12 griddlecakes
Per griddlecake: **Energy** 49 kcal / 1210 kJ
 Fat 3 g
 Fibre 0.4 g

Put the margarine and cottage cheese in a bowl and mix well. Beat in the eggs, then stir in the flour and milk and beat to a smooth thick batter.

Heat a non-stick griddle or heavy-based frying pan until very hot.

Drop tablespoons of the batter on to the hot surface. Cook for 1 minute until just set, then turn over and cook for a further 1 minute. Turn over again and continue cooking until the griddlecakes are set and golden in colour.

Transfer to a wire tray and cover with a clean cloth to keep hot while cooking the remaining batter. Serve hot with Date spread (page 121).

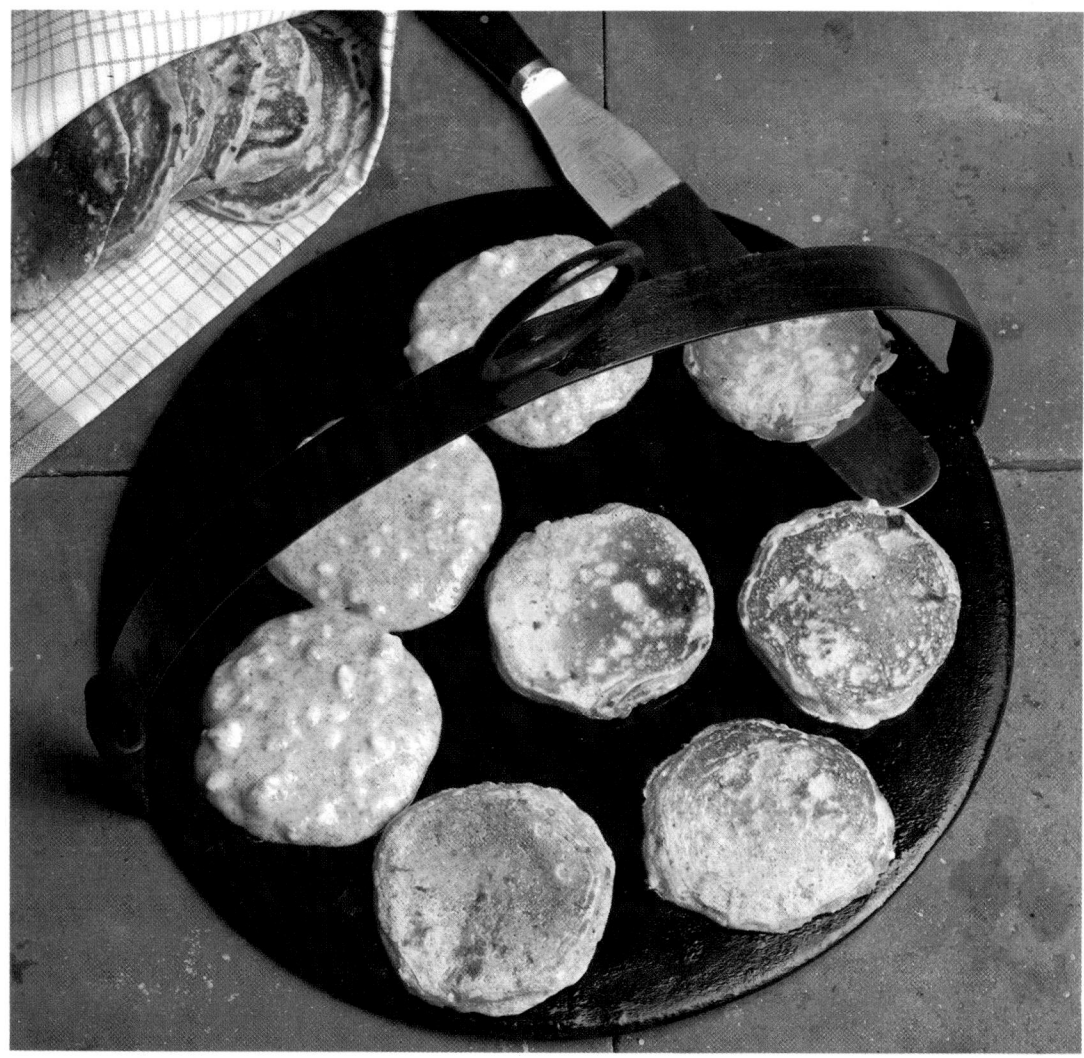

COTTAGE CHEESE GRIDDLECAKES

Desserts

APRICOT MACAROON PUDDING

225 g/8 oz dried apricots, soaked overnight in
  cold water
50 g/2 oz muscovado sugar
grated rind of ½ lemon
2 teaspoons lemon juice
MACAROONS
1 egg white
40 g/1½ oz ground almonds
40 g/1½ oz rolled oats

90 g/3½ oz caster sugar
TOPPING
25 g/1 oz flaked almonds

SERVES 6
Per serving: **Energy** 265 kcal/1120 kJ
                 Fat 8 g
                 Fibre 11 g

Cook the apricots in the soaking liquid until almost tender. Add the sugar and simmer for a further 3–4 minutes, stirring occasionally. Add the lemon rind and juice and purée in a blender until smooth.

To make the macaroons: beat the egg white until stiff, then fold in the remaining ingredients. Put the mixture into a piping bag fitted with a plain 1 cm/½ inch tube and pipe small dots on baking sheets lined with rice paper. Bake in a preheated moderate oven (180°C, 350°F, Gas Mark 4) for about 20 minutes or until lightly coloured. Cool on a wire tray, then cut off the surplus rice paper.

Arrange the macaroons in a shallow serving bowl. Spoon the apricot purée into the centre and smooth with a palette knife. Sprinkle flaked almonds on top. Place in the refrigerator for 1 hour before serving.

BAKED RAISIN CUSTARD PUDDING

4-6 slices wholemeal bread
50 g/2 oz margarine
100 g/4 oz raisins
25 g/1 oz chopped mixed candied peel
1 teaspoon grated orange rind
3-4 tablespoons demerara sugar
2 eggs

500 ml/18 fl oz skimmed milk
½ teaspoon mixed spice or ground cinnamon

SERVES 4
Per serving: **Energy** 325 kcal/1365 kJ
                 Fat 14 g
                 Fibre 5 g

Spread the bread with the margarine and cut into strips. Arrange in layers, fat-side upwards, in a 1.2 litre/2 pint ovenproof dish, sprinkling each layer with the raisins, peel, orange rind and most of the sugar. Beat the eggs and milk together and strain into the dish. Leave to stand for 15 minutes. Sprinkle with spice and then the remaining sugar. Bake in a preheated moderate oven (180°C, 350°F, Gas Mark 4) for 35-40 minutes or until set and lightly browned. Serve the pudding hot.

BAKED BANANAS WITH CHESTNUT SAUCE

6 large bananas
SAUCE
225 g/8 oz unsweetened chestnut purée
3 tablespoons unsweetened orange juice
grated rind of 1 orange
1 tablespoon lemon juice

50 g/2 oz muscovado sugar
1 teaspoon Grand Marnier (optional)

SERVES 6
Per serving: **Energy** 180 kcal/750 kJ
            Fat 1 g
            Fibre 6 g

Put the unskinned bananas on a baking sheet and bake in a preheated moderate oven (180°C, 350°F, Gas Mark 4) for about 20 minutes or until the skins are black. Remove the skins and lift the fruit carefully into a shallow serving dish. Serve the sauce separately or pour over the bananas.

For the sauce: put the ingredients in a double saucepan over hot water. Cook over a moderate heat until hot.

PEACH AND RASPBERRY CRUMBLE

225 g/8 oz dried peaches, soaked overnight in
   cold water
225 g/8 oz frozen unsweetened raspberries,
   thawed
100 g/4 oz wholemeal breadcrumbs
65 g/2½ oz muscovado sugar

SERVES 4
Per serving: **Energy** 250 kcal/1040 kJ
            Fat 1 g
            Fibre 14 g

Cook the peaches and soaking liquid for about 25 minutes or until tender. Combine the peaches and raspberries, adding enough of the liquid to make the fruit juicy.

Put the fruit into an ovenproof dish and cover with the mixed breadcrumbs and sugar. Bake in a preheated hot oven (200°C, 400°F, Gas Mark 6) for about 12 minutes or until the sugar is just caramelized and the breadcrumbs crunchy.

WINTER FRUIT SALAD

300 g/11 oz mixed dried fruits (apricots,
   prunes, peaches, apples and pears)
500 ml/18 fl oz hot, strained tea
2 tablespoons unsweetened orange juice
2 tablespoons demerara sugar
1 small lemon, thinly sliced
SAUCE
2 tablespoons desiccated coconut
1 tablespoon chopped walnuts

½ teaspoon ground ginger
2 teaspoons finely chopped stem ginger
   (optional)
250 ml/8 fl oz plain unsweetened yogurt

SERVES 4
Per serving: **Energy** 290 kcal/1220 kJ
            Fat 7 g
            Fibre 3 g

Soak the dried fruits overnight with the tea and orange juice in a 1.25 litre (2 pint) ovenproof dish. Stir in the sugar and lay the lemon slices on top. Cover with foil and cook in a preheated moderate oven (180°C, 350°F, Gas Mark 4) for 40 minutes. Discard the lemon slices.

Combine all the ingredients for the sauce and chill in the refrigerator before serving with the hot fruit salad.

SOMERSET PEARS

300 ml / ½ pint dry cider
2 strips lemon rind
1 cinnamon stick, or ¼ teaspoon ground
   cinnamon
few drops cochineal (optional)
4 dessert pears

TO DECORATE
25 g / 1 oz flaked almonds, toasted

SERVES 4
Per serving: **Energy** 90 kcal / 380 kJ
                 Fat   3 g
                 Fibre 3 g

Place the cider, lemon rind, cinnamon and cochineal, if used, in a pan. Bring to the boil, cover and boil for 1 minute.

Peel the pears carefully, without removing the stalks. Stand them upright in an ovenproof casserole, cutting a thin slice from the base of any pear which threatens to fall over.

Pour over the hot cider, cover and cook in a preheated moderate oven (180°C, 350°F, Gas Mark 4) for 30-40 minutes, basting from time to time.

Transfer the cooked pears carefully to a serving dish, and strain the liquid over them. Sprinkle with almonds and serve hot or cold.

SPICED STUFFED PEACHES

4 large peaches
1 cinnamon stick
2 whole cloves
½ teaspoon allspice berries
6 tablespoons orange juice
2-3 tablespoons brandy (optional)
FILLING
1 egg, lightly beaten

50 g / 2 oz ground almonds
1 tablespoon finely chopped stem ginger
1 tablespoon muscovado sugar

SERVES 4
Per serving: **Energy** 175 kcal / 730 kJ
                 Fat   8 g
                 Fibre 4 g

Cut the peaches in half. Remove the stones. Scoop out and reserve some of the flesh from the centre of each peach half to allow room for the filling.

To make the filling, put the egg in a bowl with the almonds, ginger, sugar and reserved peach flesh. Mix well, then spoon into the peach halves. Place the peaches in

an ovenproof dish. Scatter the spices between the fruit. Pour the orange juice over the peaches. Bake in a preheated moderate oven (180°C, 350°F, Gas Mark 4) for about 20 minutes, or until the peaches are tender when pierced with a skewer. If liked, warm the brandy, pour over the peaches and ignite. Serve hot or cold.

BANANA SURPRISE

4 medium bananas
100 g / 4 oz raspberries

SERVES 4
Per serving: **Energy** 65 kcal / 275 kJ
                 Fat   negligible
                 Fibre 4 g

Freeze the bananas in their skins for about 3 hours. Then peel the fruit and put in individual dishes with the raspberries. The bananas taste like ice cream!

RASPBERRY CHANTILLY

450 g / 1 lb raspberries
2 tablespoons Grand Marnier or other liqueur
2 egg whites
150 ml / ¼ pint plain unsweetened yogurt
grated rind of ½ lemon
1 tablespoon caster sugar
TO DECORATE
25 g / 1 oz flaked almonds, toasted

SERVES 4
Per serving: **Energy** 125 kcal / 515 kJ
Fat 4 g
Fibre 9 g

Divide the raspberries between 4 glasses and spoon over the liqueur.

Just before serving, beat the egg whites until stiff. Fold in the yogurt carefully with the lemon rind and sugar. Spoon over the raspberries and sprinkle with the almonds.

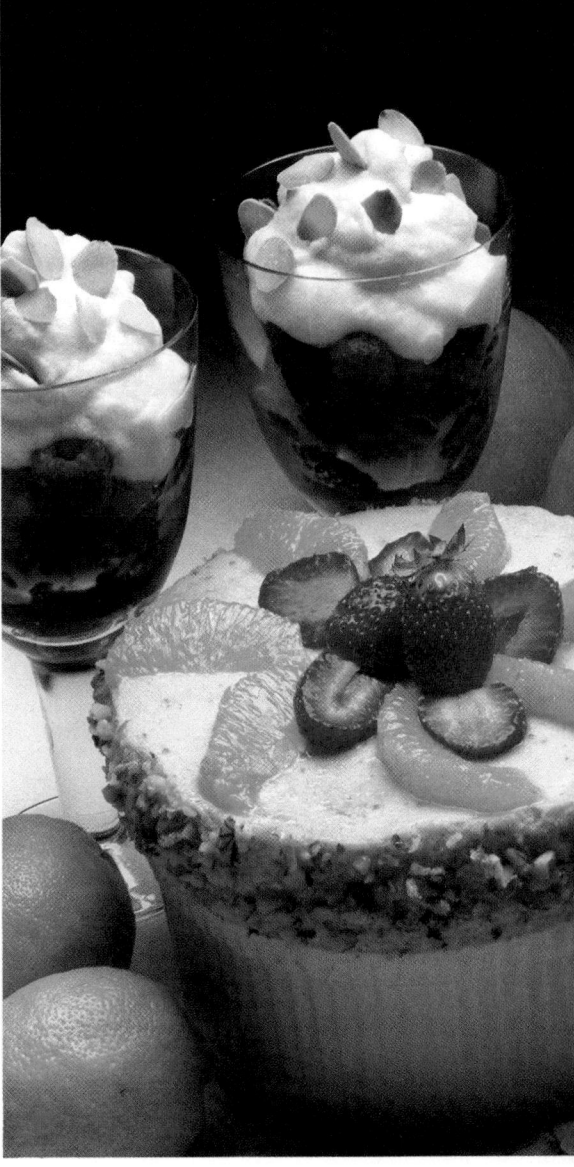

FROM LEFT: RASPBERRY CHANTILLY, STRAWBERRY AND ORANGE SOUFFLÉ, PEACH AND RASPBERRY CHEESECAKE (P. 110)

STRAWBERRY AND ORANGE SOUFFLÉ

450 g / 1 lb strawberries, hulled
4 eggs, separated
100 g / 4 oz caster sugar
finely grated rind of 1 large orange
3 tablespoons orange juice
15 g / ½ oz powdered gelatine
150 ml / ¼ pint plain unsweetened yogurt
TO DECORATE
25 g / 1 oz flaked almonds, toasted and chopped
1 orange, peeled and segmented

SERVES 6
Per serving: **Energy** 190 kcal / 805 kJ
Fat 6 g
Fibre 3 g

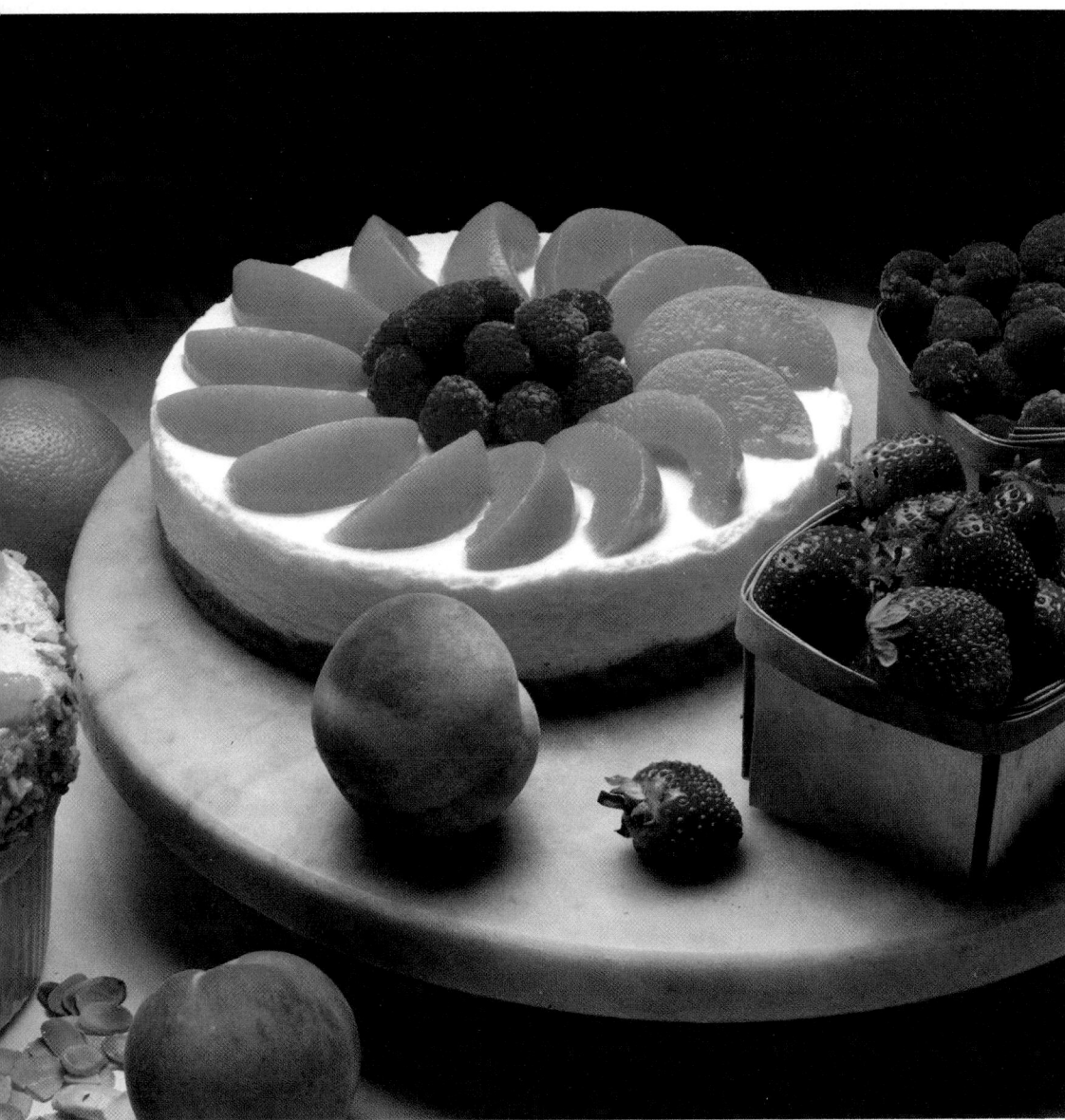

Mash the strawberries or purée in a blender, reserving a few whole ones.

Put the egg yolks in a bowl with the sugar, orange rind and half the juice. Stand the bowl over a pan of gently simmering water and whisk until the mixture is thick and pale. Remove from the heat and continue whisking until cool.

Pour the remaining orange juice into a small cup and sprinkle the gelatine on top. Stand the cup in a pan of hot water and stir until the gelatine has dissolved.

Stir the strawberry purée into the egg mixture with the yogurt and mix well. Stir in the dissolved gelatine. Leave in a cool place until thick and just beginning to set. Beat the egg whites until just stiff and fold into the mixture.

Tie a collar of greaseproof paper around a 900 ml (1½ pint) soufflé dish so that it stands 5 cm/2 inches above the rim of the dish. Pour in the soufflé mixture. Chill in the refrigerator for at least 2 hours before serving.

Remove the collar carefully before serving. Press the chopped nuts around the side. Decorate the top with the reserved strawberries and the orange segments.

PEACH AND RASPBERRY CHEESECAKE

BISCUIT CRUST
75 g/3 oz margarine
175 g/6 oz digestive biscuits, crushed
1 tablespoon demerara sugar
FILLING
350 g/12 oz cottage cheese, sieved
150 ml/¼ pint plain unsweetened yogurt
50 g/2 oz caster sugar
finely grated rind of 1 lemon
3 tablespoons lemon juice
15 g/½ oz powdered gelatine

2 tablespoons water
2 egg whites
TOPPING
2 large peaches
225 g/8 oz raspberries

SERVES 8
Per serving: **Energy** 280 kcal/1170 kJ
          Fat   14 g
          Fibre   4 g

If you do not have a loose-bottomed cake tin, make this cheesecake in an ordinary cake tin and turn it out on to a serving plate so that the crust is on top rather than underneath.

To make the crust: melt the margarine in a pan, then stir in the biscuits and sugar. Spoon the mixture into a lightly oiled 18–20 cm (7–8 inch) loose-bottomed cake tin, spread evenly and press down with the back of a spoon. Chill the crust in the tin in the refrigerator.

Meanwhile, make the filling: put the cottage cheese in a bowl with the yogurt, sugar, lemon rind and juice, reserving 1 tablespoon of lemon juice for the topping.

Beat the filling well.

Sprinkle the gelatine over the water in a small cup. Stand the cup in a pan of hot water and stir until the gelatine has dissolved. Fold into the cheese mixture.

Beat the egg whites until stiff, then fold into the cheese mixture. Pour on top of the crust in the tin and level the surface. Chill in the refrigerator until set.

To serve: run a knife around the edge of the cheesecake, then remove from the tin. Cut the peaches in half, remove the stones, then slice the flesh. Brush the cut surfaces with the reserved lemon juice. Arrange the peach slices on top of the cheesecake with the raspberries. Serve chilled. *Illustrated on p. 109.*

PEACH MOUSSE

1 tablespoon powdered gelatine
6 tablespoons hot water
1 tablespoon caster sugar
150 ml/¼ pint unsweetened peach purée (made from dried peaches)
2 tablespoons lemon juice
2 egg whites

TO DECORATE
150 ml/¼ pint plain unsweetened yogurt
chopped almonds

SERVES 4
Per serving: **Energy** 160 kcal/665 kJ
          Fat   5 g
          Fibre   4 g

Dissolve the gelatine in the hot water. Add the sugar and stir in the peach purée and lemon juice. Leave until cold and just beginning to thicken. Beat the egg whites until stiff and fold into the peach mixture. Pour into four glass dishes and chill until the mousse is set.

Just before serving, pour over the yogurt and sprinkle with chopped almonds.

VARIATION
Make the mousse as described above, using dried apricots instead of peaches to make the fruit purée.

AUTUMN PUDDING

about 10 slices wholemeal bread, crusts removed
750 g / 1½ lb dessert apples, peeled, cored and
    thinly sliced
2 tablespoons orange juice
75 g / 3 oz stoned dates, chopped
25 g / 1 oz blanched flaked almonds
1 teaspoon grated orange rind
½ teaspoon ground cinnamon (optional)

SERVES 6
Per serving: **Energy** 220 kcal / 930 kJ
                 Fat   4 g
                 Fibre 9 g

Oil the inside of a 1.25 litre (2 pint) basin lightly. Put one slice of bread in the base and overlap five more slices around the sides.

Poach the apples in the orange juice over a low heat until they are just soft. Remove from the heat. Add the dates, almonds, orange rind and cinnamon if used. Put half of this mixture into the bread-lined basin. Press another slice of bread on top. Add the remaining apple mixture. Cover the top with the remaining bread, cutting it as necessary to fit neatly. Put a small plate on top and secure this with a heavy weight. Refrigerate for 24 hours, then turn out on to a serving dish.

VARIATION
Use slices of any wholemeal fruit bread instead of plain wholemeal bread.

RHUBARB AND YOGURT FOOL

450 g / 1 lb rhubarb
2 tablespoons demerara sugar
1 tablespoon grated orange rind
1 tablespoon fresh orange juice
pinch of ground ginger
600 ml / 1 pint plain unsweetened yogurt

SERVES 4
Per serving: **Energy** 135 kcal / 590 kJ
                 Fat   2 g
                 Fibre 3 g

Cut the rhubarb into 2.5 cm / 1 inch lengths. Poach the rhubarb gently with the sugar, orange rind, orange juice and ginger until very soft. Allow it to cool.

Stir in the yogurt and chill for at least 1 hour before serving.

EXOTIC FRUIT WHIP

1 × 225 g (8 oz) can mangoes
2 egg whites, stiffly whipped
450 g / 1 lb strawberries
4 kiwi fruit, peeled and sliced

SERVES 6
Per serving: **Energy** 55 kcal / 230 kJ
                 Fat   negligible
                 Fibre 2 g

Purée the mangoes and their juice in a blender until smooth. Fold into the egg whites.

Reserve a few strawberries and slices of kiwi fruit for decoration. Place the remainder in a glass serving bowl and cover with the mango mixture. Decorate with the reserved fruit.

CHESTNUT WHIP

450 g / 1 lb chestnuts, skinned (page 36)
200 ml / ⅓ pint skimmed milk
few drops vanilla extract
finely grated rind of 1 small orange
2–3 tablespoons orange juice
2 tablespoons rum
75 g / 3 oz muscovado sugar
2 egg whites

TO DECORATE
orange twists

SERVES 6

Per serving:	Energy	205 kcal/855 kJ
	Fat	2 g
	Fibre	5 g

If fresh chestnuts are unobtainable, use one 450 g (1 lb) can unsweetened chestnut purée instead of making your own.

Put the chestnuts in a pan and add the milk and vanilla extract. Cover and cook gently for about 15 minutes until the chestnuts are soft and have absorbed the milk, stirring occasionally.

Rub through a sieve to give a thick, dry purée, then stir in the orange rind and juice, rum and sugar. Beat the egg whites until just stiff, then fold into the chestnut mixture. Spoon into a serving bowl or individual dishes or glasses. Chill in the refrigerator for at least 1 hour. Decorate with orange twists before serving.

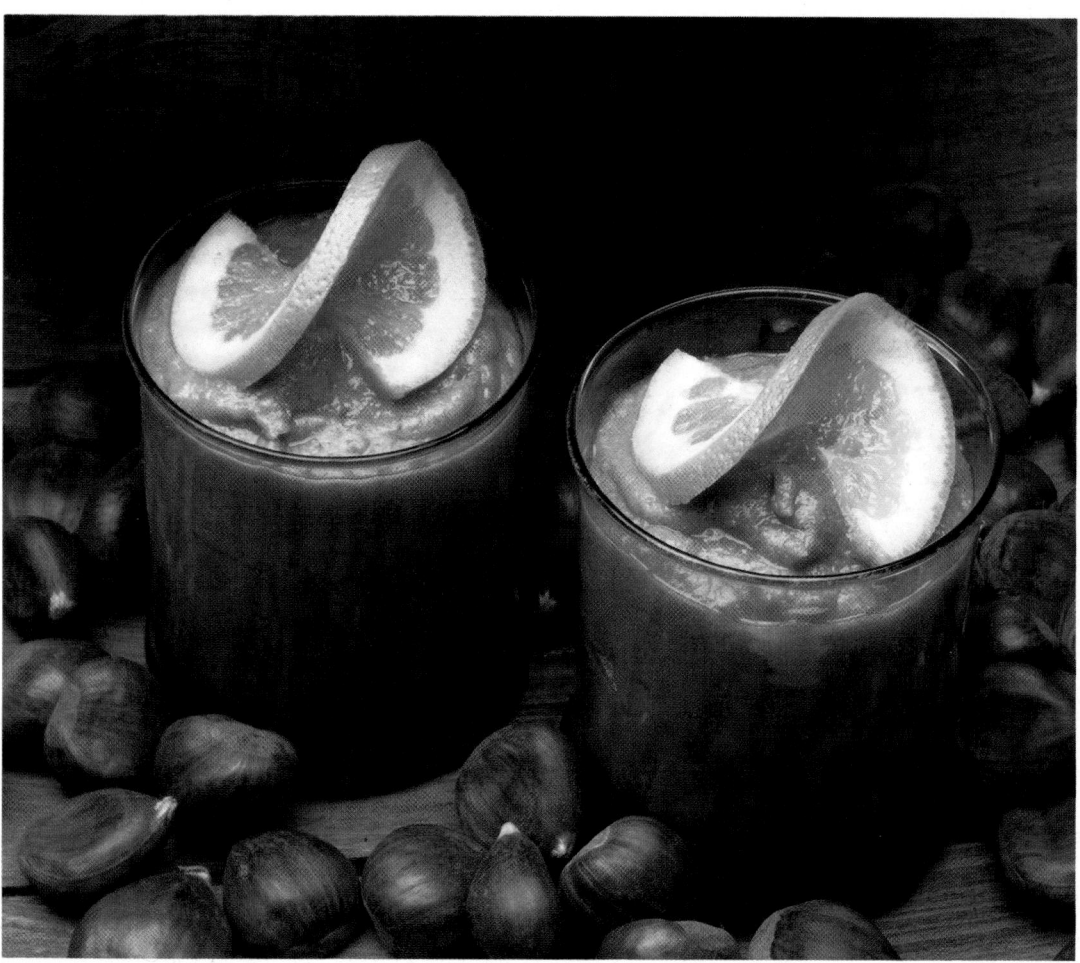

CHESTNUT WHIP

ORANGE POTS

3 tablespoons orange juice
1½ tablespoons lemon juice
1½ teaspoons powdered gelatine
350 g/12 oz quark or low-fat soft cheese
6 tablespoons buttermilk
TO DECORATE
1 orange, segmented

SERVES 4
Per serving: **Energy** 115 kcal/475 kJ
Fat 4 g
Fibre 1 g

Put the orange juice and lemon juice in a small bowl and sprinkle the gelatine on top. Stand the bowl in a pan of warm water and heat gently until the gelatine is dissolved.

Put the gelatine mixture into a blender and add the quark and buttermilk. Blend until smooth. Divide the mixture between small soufflé dishes or dessert glasses. Chill.

Decorate with orange segments shortly before serving.

GRAPE DELIGHT

450 ml/¾ pint plain unsweetened yogurt
3 egg whites

SERVES 6–8
6 servings
Per serving: **Energy** 95 kcal/400 kJ
Fat 1 g
Fibre 1 g

2 teaspoons apricot brandy (optional)
225 g/8 oz black grapes, halved and pipped
225 g/8 oz white grapes, halved and pipped

8 servings
Per serving: **Energy** 70 kcal/300 kJ
Fat 1 g
Fibre 1 g

Turn the yogurt into a bowl. Whisk the egg whites until stiff and fold into the yogurt. Stir in apricot brandy, if used.

Layer the yogurt mixture and grapes into glasses, reserving a few grapes for decoration on top of each glass.

QUARK PUDDING

dry wholemeal breadcrumbs
2 egg yolks
75 g/3 oz caster sugar
200 g/7 oz quark or low-fat soft cheese
50 g/2 oz ground almonds
1 tablespoon chopped mixed peel
3 tablespoons sultanas

2 teaspoons grated lemon rind
2 medium oranges, peeled and segmented

SERVES 8
Per serving: **Energy** 140 kcal/590 kJ
Fat 4 g
Fibre 2 g

Coat the bottom and side of a lightly oiled 15 cm (6 inch) loose-bottomed round cake tin with the breadcrumbs.

Beat the egg yolks with the sugar until pale and fluffy. Mix in the cheese, almonds, peel, sultanas and lemon rind.

Turn into the tin and smooth the top.

Bake in a preheated moderate oven (180°C, 350°F, Gas Mark 4) for about 30 minutes or until firm to the touch.

Leave to cool, then turn out the pudding. Serve with segments of fresh orange.

PRUNE MOULD

225 g/8 oz prunes, soaked overnight in 450 ml/
  ¾ pint cold water
pared rind of 1 lemon
2 tablespoons lemon juice
25 g/1 oz sugar
15 g/½ oz powdered gelatine

TO DECORATE
blanched almonds

SERVES 4
Per serving: Energy 145 kcal/620 kJ
             Fat   3 g
             Fibre   8 g

Put the prunes and soaking liquid into a saucepan. Add the lemon rind and simmer until tender.

Drain the prunes, reserving the strained liquid. Remove the stones, then purée the prunes in a blender. Add the lemon juice and sugar to the prune purée. Stir in enough of the reserved prune liquid to make the mixture up to 750 ml/1¼ pints.

Dissolve the gelatine in 2 tablespoons of the prune juice over a low heat and stir into the prune mixture. Pour into a mould and chill until set.

To serve, turn the mould out on to a serving plate and decorate with blanched almonds.

ORANGE SORBET WITH RASPBERRIES

300 ml/½ pint plain unsweetened yogurt
grated rind of 2 oranges
1 × 175 ml(6 fl oz) can frozen unsweetened
   orange juice
2 tablespoons caster sugar
2 egg whites
225 g/8 oz fresh raspberries

SERVES 4
Per serving: Energy 105 kcal/435 kJ
             Fat   1 g
             Fibre   4 g

Put the yogurt, orange rind, frozen orange juice and 1 tablespoon of the sugar into a blender and liquidize. Pour into ice cube trays and freeze for about 30 minutes. Then turn into a bowl, whisk and return to the trays. Repeat 30 minutes later. Check after a further 1½–2 hours in the freezer to see if the mixture is mushy. If so, remove from the freezer and stir in the egg whites which have been stiffly beaten with the remaining sugar. Freeze until required.

Allow to thaw for 10 minutes at room temperature before serving with the raspberries in individual bowls.

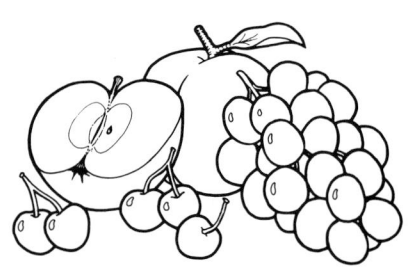

Drinks

MOCHA MILKSHAKE

175 ml/6 fl oz skimmed milk, chilled
2 teaspoons carob powder
½ teaspoon instant coffee powder
2 teaspoons unsweetened chestnut purée
1 egg white
TOPPING
1 teaspoon chopped hazelnuts

SERVES 1
Per serving: **Energy** 155 kcal/650 kJ
                Fat 6 g
                Fibre 1 g

Purée all the ingredients in a blender until thoroughly mixed and frothy. Pour into a tall glass and sprinkle hazelnuts on top.

BANANA COOLER

25 g/1 oz unsalted peanuts
175 ml/6 fl oz iced water
1 banana
1 tablespoon lemon juice
pinch of cinnamon

SERVES 1
Per serving: **Energy** 200 kcal/845 kJ
                Fat 12 g
                Fibre 5 g

Put the peanuts and 4 tablespoons of the water in a blender and purée until liquidized. Add the remaining water, the banana, lemon juice and cinnamon. Purée until smooth.

Serve the Banana cooler well chilled.

STRAWBERRY CRUSH

175 g/6 oz fresh strawberries, hulled
1–2 teaspoons caster sugar
300 ml/½ pint chilled unsweetened orange juice
ice cubes

SERVES 4
Per serving: **Energy** 50 kcal/215 kJ
                Fat negligible
                Fibre 1 g

Put the strawberries into a blender with the sugar and orange juice. Blend ½–1 minute until smooth. Serve with an ice cube in each glass.

VARIATION
Blend strawberries and sugar, divide between the glasses and fill up with chilled soda water.

APRICOT PUNCH

225 g/8 oz dried apricots, soaked overnight in
   cold water
75 g/3 oz caster sugar
250 ml/8 fl oz orange juice
2 tablespoons lemon juice
250 ml/8 fl oz dry cider
soda water, to serve
TO DECORATE
sprigs of borage or mint
glacé cherries (optional)

SERVES 8–10
8 servings

Per serving:	Energy	110 kcal/465 kJ
	Fat	negligible
	Fibre	7 g

10 servings

Per serving:	Energy	90 kcal/375 kJ
	Fat	negligible
	Fibre	5 g

Simmer the apricots and the soaking liquid with the sugar until tender. Purée the apricots and liquid in a blender until smooth. Combine the orange and lemon juice and cider in a large bowl and stir in the apricot mixture. Chill.

For each serving, fill a tumbler one-third full with apricot punch. Top with soda water and decorate with a borage or mint sprig and a cherry on a stick, if liked.

NECTARINE COCKTAIL

25 g/1 oz blanched almonds
175 ml/6 fl oz iced water
1 nectarine, stoned

SERVES 1

Per serving:	Energy	180 kcal/750 kJ
	Fat	13 g
	Fibre	6 g

Put the almonds and 4 tablespoons of the water in a blender and purée until liquidized. Add the remaining water and the nectarine. Purée until smooth. Serve chilled.

FRESH VEGETABLE COCKTAIL

2 inner celery sticks, with leaves, sliced
1 medium carrot, scrubbed and sliced
5 cm/2 inch piece cucumber, sliced
small piece red or green pepper, sliced
1 spring onion, sliced
6 large stalks watercress
450 ml/¾ pint tomato or orange juice, fresh or
   frozen
mint or basil leaves

freshly ground black pepper
150 ml/¼ pint water
ice cubes

MAKES 750 ml/1¼ pints

Total volume:	Energy	190 kcal/800 kJ
	Fat	negligible
	Fibre	4 g

Put all the vegetables into a blender with enough tomato or orange juice to cover the blades and blend for 30 seconds. Add mint leaves to orange juice; basil leaves to tomato juice. Add pepper, the remaining juice and the water and ice cubes. Blend a further 30 seconds.

Serve the cocktail as a starter or as a snack. Store in the refrigerator until required.

OPPOSITE: APRICOT PUNCH

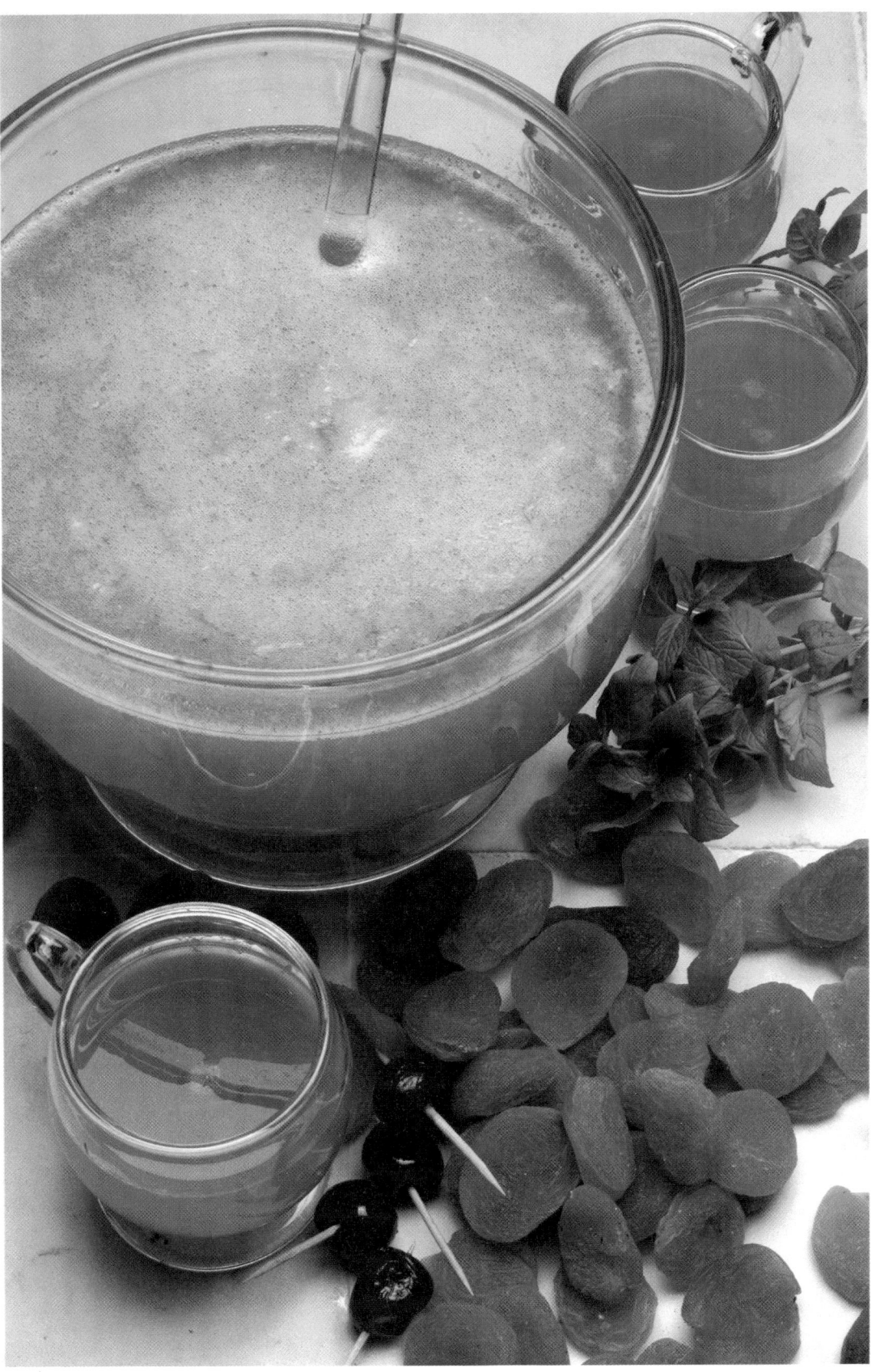

RED PEPPER COCKTAIL

450 ml / ¾ pint plain unsweetened yogurt
185 g / 6½ oz red pepper, cored, seeded and
    finely chopped
TO GARNISH
sprigs watercress

SERVES 3
Per serving: **Energy** 90 kcal / 360 kJ
                    Fat 1 g
                    Fibre 1 g

Purée the red pepper with the yogurt in a blender until smooth. Serve chilled in wine glasses. Garnish with watercress.

VARIATION
Use green pepper instead of red and garnish with finely chopped chives.

BRAZILIAN QUENCHER

25 g / 1 oz Brazil nuts
4 tablespoons iced water
1 tablespoon lemon juice
1 large orange, peeled and divided into segments

SERVES 1
Per serving: **Energy** 190 kcal / 790 kJ
                    Fat 15 g
                    Fibre 4 g

Put the nuts and water into a blender and purée until smooth. Add the lemon juice and orange segments. Purée until smooth. Serve chilled.

LEMONADE

3 lemons, scrubbed and chopped
1 tablespoon clear honey
600 ml / 1 pint iced water
TO GARNISH
2 tablespoons chopped fresh mint
water

MAKES about 750 ml / 1¼ pints
Total volume: **Energy** 65 kcal / 275 kJ
                    Fat negligible
                    Fibre 8 g

To make the garnish: pack the mint into an ice cube tray, top up with water and freeze.
   Put the lemons, honey and iced water in a blender and purée until well mixed.
   Serve the lemonade in tall glasses with iced mint cubes.

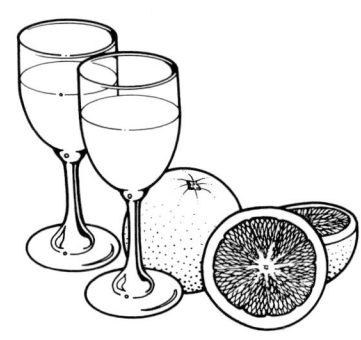

Storecupboard Recipes

PEACH MUESLI

225 g / 8 oz rolled oats
25 g / 1 oz oat bran
25 g / 1 oz wheat germ
50 g / 2 oz hazelnuts, chopped
50 g / 2 oz dried peaches, chopped
50 g / 2 oz dried apples or pears, chopped

MAKES 450 g / 1 lb
Total volume:	Energy	1445 kcal / 6075 kJ
	Fat	40 g
	Fibre	46 g

Mix all the ingredients together thoroughly and store in a glass stoppered jar.

FRESH TOMATO SAUCE

4 tablespoons olive oil
2 medium onions, chopped
2 garlic cloves, crushed
450 g / 1 lb tomatoes, chopped
1 celery stick, thinly sliced
150 ml / ¼ pint chicken stock
freshly ground black pepper

pinch of oregano or chopped fresh parsley
pinch of sugar

MAKES 900 ml / 1½ pints
Total volume:	Energy	640 kcal / 2680 kJ
	Fat	60 g
	Fibre	9 g

It is a good idea to prepare a large quantity of this sauce when tomatoes are cheaper in the autumn, then freeze it in small and large freezer bags until required.

Heat the oil in a pan and cook the onions and garlic until lightly brown. Add the tomatoes and celery and simmer gently for 5 minutes. Add the stock, pepper to taste, herbs and sugar, and continue to cook slowly for a further 10 minutes. Purée in a blender until smooth.

VARIATION
For a hotter sauce, cook one finely chopped chilli pepper with the tomatoes.

FRESH VEGETABLE SAUCE

1 red or green pepper, cored, seeded and chopped
1 medium onion, chopped
2 celery sticks, chopped
6 tomatoes, chopped
2 sprigs thyme
4 tablespoons chopped fresh parsley
freshly ground black pepper

2 garlic cloves, crushed (optional)
thin strip lemon rind

MAKES 300 ml/½ pint

Total volume:	**Energy**	70 kcal/295 kJ
	Fat	negligible
	Fibre	6 g

Put all the ingredients into a blender and blend for 1 minute. Turn out and chill.

This sauce can also be made by chopping all the ingredients very, very finely.

DAMSON SAUCE

225 g/8 oz ripe damsons, halved and stones removed
1½ tablespoons demerara sugar
2 tablespoons flaked almonds, chopped
3 × 2.5 cm (1 inch) strips orange rind
4 tablespoons orange juice

MAKES about 250 ml/½ pint

Total volume:	**Energy**	310 kcal/1305 kJ
	Fat	16 g
	Fibre	14 g

Place all the ingredients in a medium pan, bring to the boil, cover and simmer for about 5 minutes until cooked. Cool. Remove the strips of orange rind.

Place the fruit and juice in a blender and blend until a smooth purée. Serve hot or cold. This sauce can be kept in a refrigerator for 2–3 days.

CRUNCHY PEANUT BUTTER

300 g/11 oz unsalted peanuts
15 g/½ oz wheatgerm
2 teaspoons lime or lemon juice
1 teaspoon olive oil
6 tablespoons cold water
6 tablespoons sesame seeds, ground

MAKES about 350 g/12 oz

Total volume:	**Energy**	2335 kcal/9805 kJ
	Fat	100 g
	Fibre	39 g

Put the peanuts on a baking sheet and roast in a preheated moderately hot oven (200°C, 400°F, Gas Mark 6) for about 7–8 minutes or until the skins have split. Remove from the oven and rub off the skins.

Put all the ingredients in a blender and purée until thoroughly mixed. It may be necessary to beat the mixture with a wooden spoon before transferring to a screw-topped jar.

DATE SPREAD

350 g / 12 oz stoned dates
275 ml / 9 fl oz unsweetened orange juice

MAKES about 400 g / 14 oz
Total volume: **Energy** 970 kcal / 4080 kJ
Fat negligible
Fibre 30 g

Either chop the dates very finely or grind in a food mill. Then put the dates and orange juice in a saucepan. Cook over a low heat for about 5 minutes until smoothly blended.

Cool and store in the refrigerator.

QUICK DATE CHUTNEY

450 g / 1 lb stoned dates, chopped
1 small onion, finely chopped
150 ml / ¼ pint cider vinegar
1 tablespoon grated orange rind
½ teaspoon ground cloves
½ teaspoon ground mixed spice
freshly ground black pepper

MAKES about 500 g / 1¼ lb
Total volume: **Energy** 1135 kcal / 4760 kJ
Fat negligible
Fibre 40 g

Put all the ingredients into a large bowl. Mix together thoroughly until the dates have absorbed some of the vinegar. Cover and leave to marinate in the refrigerator for 24 hours.

Use the chutney within one week.

BEETROOT CHUTNEY

1.5 kg / 3¼ lb cooked beetroot, diced
750 g / 1½ lb cooking apples, cored and chopped
2 large onions, chopped
600 ml / 1 pint cider vinegar
1 teaspoon ground ginger
1½ teaspoons ground mixed spice
225 g / 8 oz demerara sugar

MAKES about 2 kg / 4½ lb
Total volume: **Energy** 1895 kcal / 7955 kJ
Fat negligible
Fibre 60 g

Put all the ingredients, except the beetroot, into a large saucepan. Bring to the boil over a low heat and cook for about 20 minutes until soft. Add the beetroot and boil for a further 10 minutes.

Put the mixture into warmed glass jars and cover it when cold.

MEAL PLANS

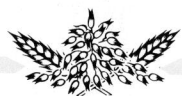

The following suggestions show how to combine different recipes to achieve high-fibre diets of varying energy levels.

The 1500 kcal/6300 kJ meal plans are suitable for people who need to lose weight. The 2000 kcal/8400 kJ and 2500 kcal/10500 kJ plans are for women and men respectively whose present weight is satisfactory; these energy levels are only guidelines since a very active person may require a higher energy intake to maintain his or her ideal weight.

1500 kcal/6300 kJ

PLAN 1

600 ml/1 pint skimmed milk

BREAKFAST
small glass fresh fruit juice
1 boiled egg
2 slices wholemeal bread or toast
thinly spread with butter or margarine
tea or coffee

LUNCH
Grapefruit tuna pâté
2 slices wholemeal bread or toast
fresh fruit

TEA
1 Carrot bun with Date spread
tea

EVENING MEAL
Prune soup
Crunchy baked bean and tomato casserole
Chicory and potato salad
Grape delight

PLAN 2

600 ml/1 pint skimmed milk

BREAKFAST
small glass fresh fruit juice
100 g/4 oz Peach muesli
tea or coffee

LUNCH
White bean salad
2 slices wholemeal bread or toast
fresh fruit

TEA
tea

EVENING MEAL
Watercress soup
Lemon mackerel
Broccoli with yogurt
100 g/4 oz baked potato with its jacket
Banana surprise

2000 kcal/8400 kJ

PLAN 1

600 ml/1 pint skimmed milk

BREAKFAST
½ grapefruit
2 slices wholemeal bread or toast with Date spread
tea or coffee

PLAN 2

600 ml/1 pint skimmed milk

BREAKFAST
small glass fresh fruit juice
2 Oatmeal muffins with quark or cottage cheese
tea or coffee

LUNCH
Wholemeal pizza
Spinach and walnut salad
fresh fruit
TEA
Strawberry crush
1 Honey and walnut scone thinly spread
  with butter or margarine
EVENING MEAL
Cucumber and yogurt soup
West African prawns and black-eye beans
100 g/4 oz brown rice
Avocado, grapefruit and sesame salad
Quark pudding

LUNCH
Spinach soup
American succotash salad
2 slices wholemeal bread
Orange sorbet with raspberries
TEA
Brazilian quencher
EVENING MEAL
Prune-stuffed tomatoes
Chinese chicken and bean-sprouts
100 g/4 oz baked potato with its jacket
Apricot macaroon pudding

2500 kcal/10500 kJ

PLAN 1
600 ml/1 pint skimmed milk

BREAKFAST
small glass fresh fruit juice
100 g/4 oz Peach muesli
1 poached egg
1 slice wholemeal toast
tea or coffee
LUNCH
Toasted turkey sandwich
1 Date and apple crunchie
fresh fruit
TEA
2 Banana drop scones
tea
EVENING MEAL
Chilled avocado soup
West Indian tuna fish risotto
Winter fruit salad

PLAN 2
600 ml/1 pint skimmed milk

BREAKFAST
small glass fresh fruit juice
2 Cornmeal waffles
tea or coffee
LUNCH
Sardinian seafood salad
2 slices wholemeal bread
1 slice Fig loaf
TEA
Banana cooler
EVENING MEAL
Stuffed artichoke – cauliflower stuffing
Peanut-stuffed chicken
Fabonade
100 g/4 oz baked potato with its jacket
Peach and raspberry cheesecake

FIBRE CONTENT OF FOODS

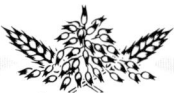

The following table shows the amount of fibre contained in some common foods. Remember that fibre is only found in foods of vegetable origin: cereals, pulses, fruit, nuts and vegetables. There is no fibre in poultry, meat, fish, cheese and other dairy products.

The fibre content is given per 100 g/4 oz of each item.

CEREALS, FLOURS AND SEEDS

bran	44 g	brown rice	4 g
100 % wholemeal flour	10 g	plain white flour	3 g
wholemeal pasta	10 g	cornmeal	2 g
oatmeal	7 g	cracked wheat	2 g
pearl barley	6 g	popcorn	2 g
sesame seeds	5 g	white rice	2 g

BREAD

100% wholemeal bread (per average slice 3 g)	8 g	white bread (per average slice 1 g)	3 g

BREAKFAST CEREALS

All–Bran	27 g	Cornflakes	11 g
Puffed Wheat	15 g	Ready Brek	8 g
Weetabix	13 g	Rice Krispies	4 g
Shredded Wheat	12 g		

BISCUITS

rye crispbread (Ryvita)	12 g	cream crackers	3 g
digestives	6 g	ginger nuts	2 g
oatcakes	4 g	shortbread	2 g

PULSES

haricot beans	25 g	peas, dried split	12 g
kidney beans	25 g	baked beans, canned	7 g
chick peas	15 g	mung beans	4 g
lentils, dried	12 g		

FRUIT

apricots, dried	24 g	currants, dried	9 g
figs, dried	18 g	dates, dried	9 g
passionfruit (skin removed)	16 g	red currants	8 g
prunes, dried	16 g	blackberries	7 g
peaches, dried	14 g	raisins	7 g
blackcurrants	9 g	raspberries	7 g

sultanas	7 g	mangoes	2 g
loganberries	6 g	nectarines	2 g
lemons, whole	5 g	oranges	2 g
cranberries	4 g	pears	2 g
damsons	4 g	plums	2 g
bananas	3 g	strawberries	2 g
gooseberries	3 g	apricots, canned	1 g
rhubarb	3 g	grapes	1 g
apples, dessert (with skin)	2 g	grapefruit	1 g
apricots, fresh	2 g	honeydew melon	1 g
avocado flesh	2 g	peaches	1 g
cherries	2 g	pineapple, fresh	1 g

NUTS (no shells)

coconut, desiccated	24 g	chestnuts	7 g
almonds	14 g	hazelnuts	6 g
Brazil nuts	10 g	walnuts	5 g
peanuts	8 g		

VEGETABLES

peas, frozen	8 g	watercress	3 g
spinach	6 g	aubergine	2 g
sweetcorn, canned	6 g	bamboo shoots	2 g
peas, fresh	5 g	cabbage, hard	2 g
vine leaves	5 g	cauliflower	2 g
broad beans	4 g	celery	2 g
broccoli tops	4 g	lettuce	2 g
Brussels sprouts	4 g	marrow and courgettes	2 g
globe artichokes	4 g	mushrooms	2 g
mustard and cress	4 g	potatoes, baked (with skins)	2 g
olives	4 g	tomatoes, fresh	2 g
parsnips	4 g	fennel	1 g
spring greens	4 g	gherkins	1 g
beansprouts	3 g	Jerusalem artichokes	1 g
beetroot	3 g	kohlrabi	1 g
cabbage, red	3 g	onions	1 g
carrots	3 g	peppers	1 g
French beans	3 g	potatoes, peeled and boiled	1 g
leeks	3 g	radishes	1 g
spring onions	3 g	tomatoes, canned	1 g
swedes	3 g	cucumber	negligible
turnips	3 g		

INDEX

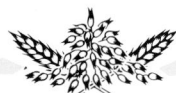